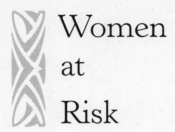

Women
at
Risk

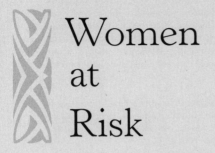

Women at Risk

THE HPV EPIDEMIC
AND YOUR CERVICAL HEALTH

Gregory S. Henderson, M.D., Ph.D.,
and Batya Swift Yasgur, M.A., MSW,

with Allan Warshowsky, M.D.

AVERY
A MEMBER OF
PENGUIN PUTNAM INC.
NEW YORK

Most Avery books are available at special quantity discounts for bulk purchase for sales promotions, premiums, fund-raising, and educational needs. Special books or book excerpts also can be created to fit specific needs. For details, write Putnam Special Markets, 375 Hudson Street, New York, NY 10014.

AVERY

a member of
Penguin Putnam Inc.
375 Hudson Street
New York, NY 10014
www.penguinputnam.com

Library of Congress Cataloging-in-Publication Data

Henderson, Gregory.
    Women at risk : the HPV epidemic and your cervical health /
Gregory S. Henderson and Batya Swift Yasgur, with Allan Warshowsky.
        p.   cm.
    Includes bibliographical references and index.
    ISBN 1-58333-128-X
    1. Papillomavirus diseases.   2. Cervix uteri—Cancer—Diagnosis.
3. Pap test.   I. Yasgur, Batya Swift.   II. Warshowsky, Allan.   III. Title.
RC168.P15H46   2002   2001056639
616.9'25'0082—dc21

Printed in the United States of America
10   9   8   7   6   5   4   3   2   1

Book design by Meighan Cavanaugh

*For my daughters, Margaux Masters Henderson
and Ava Julien Henderson*

—GSH

Contents

Acknowledgments

First and foremost, my thanks go to all of the patients who have given me the privilege of their confidence and trust. My discussions and consultations with them over the years have taught me that there is a new way to practice pathology—by directly educating people, not just about "disease," but about *their* disease. I have discovered that this educational process can be a valuable asset in a person's journey back to a state of health. And it is also personally rewarding and inspiring for me. We pathologists are so often viewed as the doctors with the bad news, so you can imagine the sense of fulfillment and joy I take in my growing collection of thank-you notes from patients. Consider this book my thank-you note back to all of you.

I have been particularly blessed with meeting many individuals who have parted the turbulent book-writing waters. With their help, I managed to cross the river without drowning during this long and daunting process of turning my dream of public education about the human papillomavirus into a book. In particular, my thanks go to Laura Shepherd and Dara Stewart, my editors at Avery. They are a pleasure to work with, wonderful and highly committed individuals. I would also like to thank Batya Swift Yasgur, not just a coauthor, but a motivator and friend as well. Many thanks to Jeffrey Celeste, superb cytotechnologist by day and graphic artist by night, for the illustrations in this book. Cristy Moore provided excellent assistance with the tedious task of reference collection and organization. My partners Warren White, M.D., and Brian Shiro, M.D., and all the incredible staff at the Women's Diagnostic Division of Wilmington Pathology Associates are to be greatly commended for their support of this project and for helping me manifest a new vision of cervical cancer screening in our area of the country. My close association with the eminent gynecologic oncologist John L. Powell, M.D., has helped me gain a deeper understanding of the nuances of cervical disease treatment.

I must thank my wife, Isabelle, for encouraging me to stop simply talking about the problem of the HPV epidemic and its impact on cervical health and to start writing about it instead, and for her love, support, and intense critique during the process. My father, Julian C. Henderson, M.D., still the best pathologist I know, has been a great source of historical perspective in this work, and continues in his retirement to fight the good fight against the "commodification" of the Pap smear. My mother, my sisters, and my closest friends have participated in some way in this work through words of encouragement and manuscript critique. No simple words of thanks can express how much of this book is a reflection of their love for me and mine for them.

—GSH

Introduction

Most people have never heard of the human papillomavirus, or HPV, even though its prevalence is far greater than the much-talked-about human immunodeficiency virus (HIV). Public health officials have done a splendid job educating the population about HIV, including what it is, how it's transmitted, and what can be done to prevent it, which has helped in lowering the transmission of this virus. In contrast, your chances of becoming infected or of already being infected with HPV are one in two. The fact is, human papillomavirus is now the number-one sexually transmitted disease (STD) and the number-one cause of cervical cancer in America and the rest of the world.

For most people, the idea that cancer can be caused by a virus is almost completely unknown. Cancer has for so long been the great "mystery disease" of our advanced medical society—much like infectious diseases were during the nineteenth century. Although medicine has made some phenomenal advances in the understanding of how cancers develop—particularly in the past ten years—we still don't know the actual cause of most cancers. But, as unbelievable as it sounds, we *do* now know that some cancers—those of the vagina, cervix, and vulva—are caused by a viral infection.

The sad fact is that the medical and scientific community has known that HPV is the culprit in these cancers of women for about ten years. "We" have done a great job of designing new tests and modifying old ones to catch this culprit at work earlier and earlier, but we have done a terrible job of informing *you* about HPV.

A painfully unjust reality of HPV infection is that the majority of actual disease resulting from infection occurs in women. As I will discuss later, men can suffer from some of the ill effects of the virus and certainly can carry and transmit it, but women, by far, bear the heaviest burden of disease. For this reason, much of the focus of this book will be about the manifestations, detection, and treatment of disease in women. But make no mistake, this is a sexually transmitted disease of both women and men, and in my opinion, men should be as informed about this insidious virus as women so that they can take the appropriate measures to protect themselves and the women with whom they are involved from these diseases.

There is plenty of good news, however, and the mission of this book is to tell you about positives, not just negatives. The fact is that although at least half of us may be infected with HPV in our lifetime, only a very small percentage of women develop precancerous changes that require treatment and even fewer women develop full-blown cervical cancer. We now know quite a bit about which specific types of HPV are most associated with the development of cancer. In addition, the diagnostic tests designed to discover high-risk types of HPV and very early cancerous changes have improved dramatically. This has allowed us to catch these cancers early and effectively cure the majority of them.

Perhaps the best news of all is that you are reading this book, which is designed to educate you (and hopefully everyone you know) about this virus—how it is transmitted, what strategies you can use to prevent it, and what your options are if you are suffering from some of its effects.

How Prevalent Is HPV?

Human papillomavirus is actually a family of viruses, and more than 100 members have now been identified. You are probably familiar with the virus even if you've never heard the name because many of its family members cause the common wart that we most often see on hands and feet. Fairy-tale witches with nasty cackles and warty noses have been infected by HPV. Some members of the HPV family specifically infect the genital tracts. These genital strains of HPV are the subject of this book.

Genital HPV infection is alarmingly on the rise, especially in the United States and other developed countries. In many areas of the world, it is an even more serious problem, with cervical cancer being more common than breast cancer in areas such as Central and South America. Almost 99 percent of all cervical cancers are related to HPV infection. According to the Centers for Disease Control, there are 45 million cases of undetected HPV in the United States, and current data indicate that 60 to 80 percent of people will be infected by HPV in their lifetime. Most recent statistics show that 12,800 American women contract cervical cancer every year. Worldwide, about 320,000 women, 4,800 of whom are American, still die of this preventable disease every year. Sadly, a less recognized issue is the astounding number of long-term effects that HPV-related disease causes. Even more disturbing is the fact women and young girls are contracting the virus at increasingly earlier ages, since the age of sexual activity is becoming progressively younger.

The implications of these statistics and trends are staggering. With the rapid increase in the spread of the virus, we are seeing dramatic increases in the incidence of HPV-related disease. And remember that all of these alarming trends are set against a backdrop of a near complete lack of public awareness of this virus.

WHY I WROTE THIS BOOK

I am a pathologist with a busy practice that spans a large portion of North Carolina. I specialize in cancers of women, which means that I spend a great deal of time every day diagnosing diseases related to HPV infection.

I often find that people know as much or as little about pathology as they do about HPV. Most people associate pathologists with those who perform autopsies—the white-coated figures in mystery novels, revealing to the detective some vital clue regarding the death of the murder victim. But this unfortunate (and rather morbid) association focuses on only a tiny fraction of what pathologists actually do. In reality, the specialty of pathology is broadly the specialty of diagnostic medicine. The majority of my time is spent looking through the microscope making diagnoses from either biopsies or major surgical excisions; interacting with surgeons in the operating room and guiding surgical procedures by making rapid, so-called "frozen-section" diagnoses; and running the clinical laboratory that performs millions of diagnostic tests per year. In short, every time you have a biopsy or blood taken by another physician, the specimen is sent to a pathologist, who examines and interprets the slide or runs the test and communicates his or her findings to your doctor, often with recommendations for treatment. This doesn't leave a lot of time for solving murder mysteries.

One of my most important roles as a pathologist is looking at Pap smears, samples of the cervix taken by gynecologists during examination. I spend a good portion of my day peering through a microscope lens at slides of abnormal smears. These are screened and flagged as abnormal by my excellent staff of *cytotechnologists*—highly trained experts who specialize in the screening and detection of microscopic cellular abnormalities. Based on these slides, I can usually determine whether a woman is suffering from some precancerous or cancerous cervical condition. The woman's gynecologist then uses this information, together with visual examination, to implement a course of treatment.

As much as I love and am challenged by my specialty, I have never been content merely with pushing glass slides under a microscope and generating a computerized lab report for the patient and her gynecologist. Every specimen I examine comes from a person who is, more often than not, waiting anxiously to find out what is wrong and usually really wants to understand her disease. So, I often take the rather unconventional step of meeting with patients, usually women, by virtue of my subspecialty, who want to discuss what the diagnosis means and how it relates to various treatment options. I try to alleviate fears and provide education regarding prevention of future problems.

THE STORY OF KATE

"Tell them my story, Dr. Henderson. I had never heard of this HPV. I didn't know about what could happen to me. I didn't know that cervical cancer is caused by an STD. I'm going to die, but maybe my story can save other women."

These are the words of a patient I'll call Kate, who died of cervical cancer at the age of thirty-two. She had been a normal teenager, experimenting with sex—although in a more limited way than many other teens I've worked with—but she eventually developed a stable relationship with one young man who ultimately became her boyfriend.

Kate was a healthy, vibrant young woman with no medical problems. She had never been taught about preventive care and neglected to have an annual Pap smear. At the age of twenty-nine, she consulted her gynecologist because she had begun to bleed after having intercourse. Her gynecologist examined her and immediately performed what is known as a cone biopsy. (You will learn more about that in Chapter 6.) It turned out that Kate had invasive cervical cancer. It had already spread to her lymph nodes.

After being diagnosed, Kate's first response was typical: "Why me?" She went through an anguished emotional process that was also practical. She really wanted to understand how she had contracted this disease. In the course of her explorations, she spoke to an old high school classmate who had relocated to another state. The two women had not been in touch since their senior year of high school. It turned out that her friend was also suffering from invasive cervical cancer. Kate began to understand that she and her friend had probably both contracted HPV (which I had told her about) from the same boy. Now, ten years later, she was paying the price of not knowing that the virus exists, what impact it can have, how to monitor its progress, and how to prevent its devastating consequences. She was pained and baffled by the lack of information. "Why didn't someone tell us about this illness?" she asked.

Before she died, Kate urged me to inform the public about HPV. Kate's request provided the final inspiration to complete the daunting task of writing this book. The inspiration had long been germinated by my conversations with hundreds of women diagnosed with various stages of cervical disease or other HPV-related illnesses. These women range in age from young teens to women in their seventies. As I said above, frighteningly, the age of onset is getting younger all the time, and it is now very common for such conversations to be initiated by mothers of young teens who are suffering some extreme manifestations of HPV infection. My patients come from all walks of life and all socioeconomic backgrounds. They all have one thing in common beyond the presence of cervical, vaginal, or vulvar disease: None of them had any idea of what caused their condition until I explained it to them. All these women were suffering from HPV, yet none had heard of it.

I asked colleagues across the country about their experiences with patients and found that my patients are by no means unique and that my perceptions are accurate. My fellow physicians reported that few patients had ever heard of HPV, and none knew about its connection to cervical cancer. Further research convinced me that this is a sadly neglected area of public health, and that American women need to be educated. This book is designed to provide that education. You will hear me say throughout this book that cervical cancer *is* preventable. Today, there is no reason why any woman should die of or even contract cervical cancer. I truly believe that I and others in my profession can help eradicate deaths and most long-term effects caused by HPV during my lifetime. But as we have learned with breast cancer, AIDS, and tobacco use, it can't happen without the education and participation of everyone affected.

WHO CAN BENEFIT FROM THIS BOOK?

This book is designed to teach you about HPV and the major diseases that it causes. As you may have gathered, the most serious disease caused by HPV is cervical cancer, so a large majority of this book will focus on cervical health and disease. As HPV is a sexually transmitted virus, every sexually active woman needs to be educated regarding care of her cervix and prevention of HPV. Mothers, school nurses, and others who work with teenagers need information so that they can counsel girls in the prevention of HPV. Women need to learn how to prevent the spread of an STD and about lifestyle changes (such as quitting smoking) that minimize risk of developing cervical cancer if you have been infected with HPV. And perhaps most important of all, women need to be informed about the necessity of the annual Pap smear as a screening device to provide early detection of potential problems.

If you have already been diagnosed with an HPV-induced disease such as genital warts, this book will help you understand your condition and what you can do about it. If you have received an abnormal Pap smear result, this book can help you understand what the findings mean and what your options are.

This book will also be useful for you if you are the family member of a woman with cervical disease. The information provided here is especially important for the partner of a woman diagnosed with HPV or with cervical disease. It will enable them to give their partner moral support and also to take precautions to prevent themselves from being affected by the disease.

First, you will learn in detail about the members of the family of human papillomavirus that infect the male and female genitalia, how they invade the body, and the various effects that they can have on the genitals. You will find out what cervical cancer is, how it progresses, and its connection to HPV.

In Chapter 5, you'll be introduced to the Pap smear. Once you understand what it is, how it's interpreted, and what the test results mean, you'll be ready for Chapter 6, which addresses what to do if you have an abnormal Pap smear. Chapter 7 looks at the various types of cancer that can be caused by HPV, what treatments are available, and what you can expect from each. In Chapter 8, you will find out about other diseases caused by HPV.

If you are suffering from HPV or from any cervical disease and you are thinking of having a baby, you are probably wondering how your condition will affect your chances of becoming pregnant, of carrying the baby safely to term, and of having a healthy child. Also, since HPV is a sexually transmitted disease, you may wonder how it will affect the man in your life. Chapter 9 will discuss these issues.

Chapter 10 is written by holistic gynecologist Allan Warshowsky, M.D. He is the director of the women's health program at the Continuum Center for Health and Healing of Beth Israel Hospital in New York City. Dr. Warshowsky tells you about your many treatment options if you have been diagnosed with HPV infection. He presents an array of effective conventional and complementary approaches that will help you remain symptom-free. These approaches may also help in the treatment of genital warts, cervical dysplasia, and cervical cancer. The concluding chapters provide information on preventing infection with HPV and the role you can play in preventing or curtailing the spread of this virus on a national level.

Near the end of the book, you will find suggestions for further reading, as well as a list of Internet Web sites and other resources to help you further your understanding of the topics covered in this book. There will also be a list of organizations and self-help groups you can contact for additional information and emotional support.

Cervical cancer can be prevented and the tide of the HPV epidemic can be turned. Reading this book can be a first step. I wish you good health and healing.

1

Human Papilloma *What?*

When I meet a patient newly diagnosed with HPV, the first reaction is usually a blank stare, followed by the inevitable question "Human papilloma what?" This chapter will tell you a little bit about this "new" virus—what it is, how you get it, and what it can do to you.

I put the word *new* in quotation marks because there is a very good chance that you had never heard of HPV before you picked up this book and you might be wondering whether it is a new virus, or an old one that scientists had only recently discovered. It is in fact neither. HPV is certainly a very ancient virus. Human papillomaviruses seem to have been around for as long as there have been humans to infect. Indeed, the papillomaviruses in general have found a broad niche over the last several million years of evolution, as almost every "higher" species has a group of papillomaviruses that infect it specifically.

HPV is also not a newly discovered virus. In fact, of all the viruses that have been discovered during the twentieth century, the HPV family was among the first described. In addition, Ancient Greek medical writings recognize that genital warts were sexually passed from one person to another. In 1842, an Italian physician, Rigoni-Stern, noted that cervical cancer was very common among married women and rare in nuns and unmarried women. This observation suggested to him the possibility that cervical cancer was somehow linked to sexual activity, generally thought to have been confined to marriage. In the early twentieth century, it was also observed that second wives of men whose first wife had died of cervical cancer had a much higher incidence of developing cervical cancer themselves. Again, this fueled the idea that the cancer was caused by some transmissible agent. The only piece of missing information was the name and nature of that agent.

By the time I took my first pathology course in medical school in 1986, we were familiar with a number of viruses and had come to believe that cervical cancer was caused by some sexually transmitted disease. At that time, the favored culprit was the genital herpes simplex virus (HSV). At about the same time, a revolution in DNA analysis technology was launched. New scientific understanding of this molecule made DNA a household word. Using these new techniques, it became possible not only to identify criminals based upon DNA samples, but also to pull the DNA out of a cancer cell, look at what had gone wrong with it, and search for the presence of some viral DNA that might be causing the problem. Over the next few years, through research and some quite sophisticated epidemiological and statistical analysis, scientists concluded that the culprit was not HSV but HPV.

THE HPV FAMILY TREE

HPV is actually not one single virus; rather, it's a family of viruses. Scientists have now identified about 130 members or strains of this family. Each virus is assigned a number according to the order in which it was discovered. Not the most creative "naming" system, but then again, science is not usually known for its verbal creativity. It has been found that certain strains of the virus prefer to infect certain parts of the body—although, as you will see, there is some degree of crossover. Similarly, there is considerable variety in the types of disease that they can produce, ranging from no noticeable disease to typical warts to flat warts to cancer. The following are some of the major players in the family, the sites of the body they prefer, and the diseases that they are most associated with. Most other strains rarely cause significant disease.

CONDITION	MOST COMMON HPV STRAIN
Plantar (soles of feet) warts	1
Common raised and flat warts at other skin sites	2, 3, 19, 27
Warts and cancers around and under the fingernails and toe nails (subungual digital)	16
Genital warts	2, 6, 11, 16
Laryngeal and upper airway warts (papillomas) and cancers	6, 11, 16, 18, 35
Cervical, vaginal, vulvar, penile, and anal cancers	6, 10, 11, 16, 18, 26, 31, 33, 35, 39, 45, 51, 52, 55, 56, 58, 59, 66, 68
Oral cancers	16, 18, 36, 57

It is not entirely clear what makes some viral types "prefer" different areas of the body, but part of the story lies on the surface of the virus itself, which is covered with "keys," or *ligands*. These are designed to fit the "locks" in your cell—your *cell receptors*. Ligands are very specific and can enter only receptors that fit. So the HPV strain that causes plantar warts on the feet has ligands that will link up only to skin cells on the foot with those particular receptors. This is why it is unlikely that you would contract cervical disease if your partner had a plantar wart that somehow came into contact with your genital area. The virus that likes feet does not have ligands to fit vaginal or cervical squamous cell receptors. But if you refer to the chart above, you'll notice that there are some viruses that appear able to infect multiple sites. For instance, HPV type 16, one of the major cancer causers, can infect the squamous and glandular cells of the cervix, the squamous cells of the anus, the squamous cells of the mouth, and less commonly, the fingernails and toenails. Contrast this with HPV type 1, which seems to have little to no ability to cause cancer and is found almost exclusively in warts on the soles of the feet.

From this myriad of family members, scientists have been able to further divide the viral types into two major groups—those that are more likely to cause cancer (*high-risk,* or *oncogenic, viral types*) and those that rarely lead to cancer (*low-risk viral types*). The high-risk types include 16, 18, 31, 33, 35, 38, 45, 51, 52, 56, 58, 59, and 68. The low-risk types include 6, 11, 42, 43, and 44.

HOW HPV IS TRANSMITTED

The human papillomaviruses infect primarily the surface cells of your body, including those covering the skin, mouth, esophagus, upper airways, urethra, anus, vagina, and ectocervix. They are transmitted by skin-to-skin contact. Warts on the fingers can be communicated to other fingers, and warts on the feet can be transmitted to other feet. Infections in the genital area can be communicated to other regions of the genital tract and also to the genital tract of a sexual partner. This is why we call HPV a sexually transmitted disease.

Each virus has its own mode of transmission. Chickenpox and the common cold, for example, are airborne. If you breathe the air of someone who has the virus, you can also catch it. HIV is transmitted through the exchange of body fluids. It is considered a sexually transmitted disease because during sex there is an exchange of body fluids. HPV is transmitted through skin-to-skin contact, obviously a central aspect of the sexual experience. Thus HPV can be transmitted through foreplay and "fooling around," not merely through intercourse. We will discuss this at much greater length in Chapter 4.

WHAT HAPPENS NEXT?

After the virus has infected the genital area, it might not cause you any trouble for a long time. In fact, you might not even know it's there. Unlike a cold, with which you immediately start sneezing and blowing your nose, or chickenpox, in which blisters erupt a predictable number of days after you have been exposed to the virus and infected by it, HPV can hang around for years doing nothing. Needless to say, this is a complicating and often confusing characteristic of HPV infection. Just as disturbing, the symptoms can go away, only to reappear years later. That's because the virus has not been eliminated from the system, but merely subdued. It has become dormant and can flare up at any time—especially during periods of stress, or as a result of aging.

This has *extremely* important implications when it comes to your relationship with your partner. It is crucial for you to understand that a diagnosis of an HPV-related illness is *not* immediate evidence that your partner has been unfaithful. When a patient diagnosed with HPV finds out that the virus is a sexually transmitted disease, she might react with rage, assuming that her partner has been cheating on her. But when I ask her to be absolutely honest about her own sexual history, she may realize that a sexual encounter of some sort, often many years earlier, might be the source of infection. I say "encounter" because as mentioned above, the virus is transmitted through skin-to-skin contact and can be communicated even without full-fledged intercourse. Likewise, her partner may be carrying the virus, caught many years earlier during some sexual liaison that predated his relationship with the patient. So if you're diagnosed with HPV, don't run home with divorce papers. The same is true for a flare-up. If you or your partner suddenly has a return of HPV symptoms after years of symptom-free existence, don't assume that someone has been fooling around. What's insidious about this virus is that it can lie latent and undetected for long stretches of time—sometimes for decades.

By now you might be both alarmed and confused. A virus you've never heard of might be hiding in your cells, just waiting to jump out. It can cause problems that range from genital warts to cancer. How does this happen? What goes on in the cells to allow the virus in, and how can you prevent it from doing damage if you are infected? The next chapters will help you understand what happens to the body on a cellular level when any virus—including HPV—invades, and how HPV in particular does its nasty work. You will also learn when and how HPV can cause cells to become cancerous. Chapter 11 will give you tips for prevention and for symptom reduction if you have already been infected.

2

The Ins and Outs of the
Female Reproductive System

When I was in medical school, my first course was anatomy. I'm not alone—all medical schools begin their extensive curriculum with lessons in how the body is structured and how it functions. It is impossible to know what can go wrong with the human body without first knowing how it is put together and how it functions when it works right. In other words, we must understand health before we can understand disease. In keeping with this time-honored philosophy, this chapter will be devoted to a tour of the reproductive system from the outside in—from the level of what you see with your own eyes, all the way down to what you need a microscope to see. Since the majority of actual disease resulting from HPV infection occurs in women, and because the anatomic regions of women that are most specifically targeted by the virus are rather complex, this tour will focus on female anatomy in general and specifically on the anatomy of the cervix.

THE FEMALE REPRODUCTIVE SYSTEM

The female reproductive tract is shaped like a Y, as Figure 2.1 depicts. At the top of each of the prongs of the Y sit the *ovaries*. The ovaries are small, somewhat egg-shaped organs that store the eggs, or oocytes, until they are released—usually one at a time, at one-month intervals. They also produce estrogen, the major female sex hormone.

The ovaries are connected to the uterus on either side by the fallopian tubes, which are located approximately five inches below the

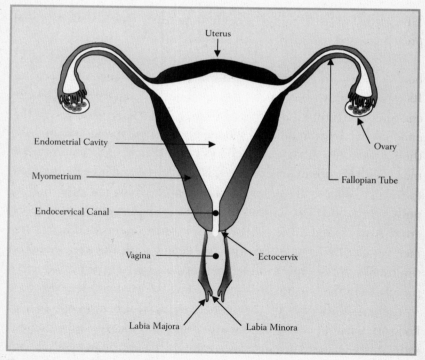

FIGURE 2.1 THE FEMALE GENITAL TRACT

waist. The fallopian tubes are named for the great sixteenth-century Italian anatomist Fallopius of Modena, without whom we would not have much to talk about in this chapter. He worked out the entire anatomy of the female reproductive system. The tubes that now bear his name are actually pretty complicated. They are best described as long thin funnels, wider at the end that attaches to the ovary than at the opposite end that enters the uterus. At the wide end of the tube are several fingerlike projections, which are designed to catch the eggs released by the ovary and to move them inside the tube for the journey to the uterus. Inside the tube, there are many more fingerlike projections and channels, which move the egg on its way. The moment of conception—when an egg is fertilized by sperm—actually occurs in the tube, so the tube must provide a good environment for sperm and for the fertilized egg in its early hours of life. If any of the tubes' many duties malfunction, the fertilized egg may not survive, or occasionally, it may implant itself and grow within the tube. This is called a tubal pregnancy, and can be a serious medical problem.

The *uterus* is shaped rather like an inverted old-fashioned Coke bottle. The central cavity of the uterus is called the *endometrial cavity.* Its wall is made of very thick muscle (about an inch thick) called *myometrium.* A fertilized egg should ultimately implant itself inside the endometrial cavity and begin growing into a fetus. As the fetus grows, the myometrium relaxes, allowing the uterus to get bigger to accommodate the growing fetus. At the time of labor, these muscles contract to push the baby into the outside world. This contractile ability is also put to use in the absence of pregnancy every month to help the old endometrial lining to be pushed out of the uterus at the end of the menstrual cycle. The menstrual cramps most women experience at this time is actually the contraction of myometrium, a mini-version of the contraction pains felt during childbirth.

The opening or "neck" of the bottle is the *cervix;* in fact, cervix is Latin for neck. For most of a woman's life, the cervix serves as a tight muscular seal that acts as a selective barrier to, or "gatekeeper" of, the uterus. It has two basic purposes—to keep invaders such as bacteria and viruses out and to keep fetuses in. Like many other muscles of the reproductive tract, the cervical muscles can expand and contract. As a rule, these muscles are clamped tightly together, leaving an opening that is no larger than four to five millimeters in diameter—slightly smaller than the diameter of a pencil. This opening is called the *os,* which is Latin for mouth, and the connection or tunnel to the uterus is called the *endocervical canal,* or the *endocervix.*

When hormones produced by the ovaries, pituitary gland, and other glands instruct them to do so, the cervical muscles relax, resulting in a widening of the os and endocervical canal. This occurs during menstruation, to allow blood and endometrial tissue to pass through. During sexual intercourse, the cervix opens to allow sperm to pass through and enter the uterus. And of course, during labor, this tight muscular gatekeeper relatively rapidly (although certainly not rapidly enough for the woman in labor) relaxes, opening from a diameter of 4 to 5 millimeters to 10 centimeters, and allows a baby and the placenta to pass through, and then promptly closes the gate again.

The cervix connects to the *vagina,* a relatively smooth mucosa-lined passageway that is generally very narrow, but stretches wide enough to allow a baby to pass through. The opening of the vagina leads to the external genital area, called the *vulva.* The vulva is divided broadly into the inner *labia minora* (Latin for "small lips") and the outer *labia majora* (Latin for "large lips"). The area where the labia minora meet the most external portion of the vagina is called the *vestibule.* The labia minora meet at the front of the vulva, covering the *clitoris,* a small, sensitive projection analogous to the penis. Where they meet at the back of the vulva, near the anus is called the *posterior fourchette* (French for "fork"). The labia majora are covered by skin and pubic hair.

A CLOSER LOOK

The reproductive tract, like all surfaces of the human body, external and internal, is covered by a layer of cells called *epithelium.* There are different types of epithelia, and which type lines which part of the body depends on the organ's function. There are two general types of cells that line the reproductive tract—*squamous* and *glandular* cells. (See Figure 2.2.)

Squamous cells are like armor. They are tough and hard to penetrate. Their purpose is to protect what's inside from invaders that are outside. They are flat and dense, adhere tightly to each other, and are good at providing a barrier against invading organisms and trauma. The skin, for example, is covered by squamous cells. Glandular cells secrete substances into the body and are also sort of porous, in that they allow necessary substances from the body to pass through into the organs. The digestive tract, for example, is covered by glandular

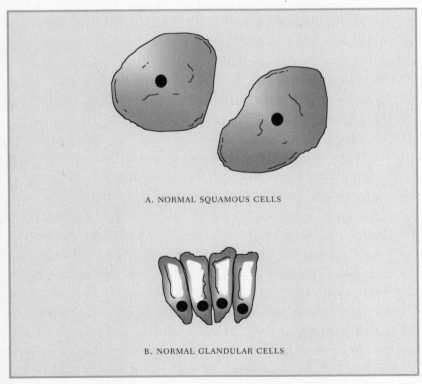

A. NORMAL SQUAMOUS CELLS

B. NORMAL GLANDULAR CELLS

FIGURE 2.2

cells. They secrete digestive juices to help break your food down so that it can be digested. They also allow the nutrients that you need to be absorbed into your body.

Squamous cells look like flat, long, thin tiles. They have a small nucleus, usually in the center, and lots of cytoplasm. Glandular cells are also called columnar cells due to their shape. At the bottom of the column sits the nucleus, and at the top of the column, the cytoplasm stores its secreting substance. In the female genital tract, almost all of the columnar cells release lubricants; nutrients for eggs, sperm, and embryos; and other compounds that help protect against infectious organisms.

The columnar cells usually stand in one layer along a basement membrane. Squamous cells, in contrast, lie on top of one another, layer upon layer. (See Figure 2.3.) This provides an extra degree of protection. Under the basement membrane lie all of the blood vessels, nerves, muscles, and connective tissue that hold an organ together and give it shape. The whole covering made of the epithelium, whether composed of glandular or squamous cells, and the basement membrane is called the mucosa. Everything under the basement membrane is called the submucosa.

It is important to remember that these epithelial squamous and glandular cells are living organisms and are subject to the same rules as all other living things—they are born, they mature, they perform their function, and they die. This cycle of cellular birth, life, and death is repeated continuously many times a day at all sites of your body that are covered by epithelial cells. All of your bodily surfaces are continuously being renewed by a new covering of cells. We can all appreciate that this is a pretty effective design because these epithelial cells are in direct contact with the outside world and are therefore the most likely to be damaged or to wear out. While the process is somewhat different for squamous and glandular epithelium, the basics are the same. Both types of epithelium contain a relatively small population of cells that are actually dividing or giving birth to new cells on the basement membrane.

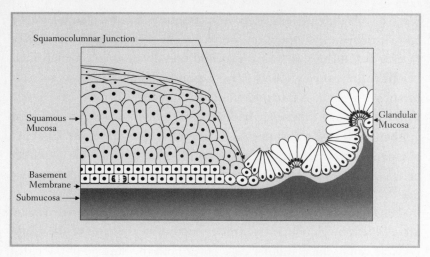

Squamocolumnar Junction

Squamous → Mucosa

Glandular → Mucosa

Basement Membrane →

Submucosa →

FIGURE 2.3 SQUAMOUS AND GLANDULAR LINING

In squamous epithelium, after a new cell is generated from this division, one of the cells stays on the basement membrane, while the other stops dividing and begins to *differentiate*—grow up and start doing its job as a squamous cell. This means it starts flattening itself out, attaching itself to the other cells around it very tightly, shrinking its nucleus (because it really doesn't need to do much thinking anymore, and it saves space), and filling up its cytoplasm with keratin, which makes the cell hard. This process of differentiation occurs as the new cell moves up the layer of tiles that forms the squamous epithelium. So, the squamous cells at the very top layers are the most differentiated. They are flat, hard tiles of keratin with a shriveled and shrunken nucleus. They are firmly anchored to the cells around them, forming a strong barrier. The squamous cells at the very bottom, still on the basement membrane, have a much larger nucleus, are still dividing, and don't have much keratin in their cytoplasm. In the middle are the cells still in the process of differentiating. When these middle cells reach the top, the current top layer will die and be shed, and the bottom level of cells will move up to the middle.

In glandular epithelium, there is a minor population of cells called reserve cells that are sprinkled throughout the mature glandular cells and sit right next to them on the basement membrane. Each time a reserve cell divides, it forms a second non-dividing cell, which then begins to grow up and do its job as a glandular cell. It fills up its cytoplasm with cervical mucus and starts squeezing it into the outside world. The major difference between the squamous and the glandular epithelium is that this process of glandular cell maturation is not accompanied by a trip up many levels of cells. Instead, all glandular cells remain on the basement membrane and don't pile up on top of one another.

The fallopian tubes, endometrial cavity, and the endocervical canal are all lined by glandular/columnar mucosa. In the case of the endocervical canal, the glandular cells cover both the surface of the canal and a number of glands that are located under the surface of the canal. These cervical glandular cells perpetually release a substance called cervical mucus, which is designed to keep the vagina moist and lubricated. It also acts as an antibiotic, killing invading bacteria before they can do any damage. It even contains chemicals that promote the transfer of sperm into the uterus. Properly functioning glandular cells continually release this mucus into the cervix and vagina.

The outer portion of the cervix—or *ectocervix*—the vagina, and the vulva are all covered by squamous mucosa. This makes sense, as squamous mucosa is more protective. Bacterial invaders and other toxins are likely to enter the system through the outside. Plus, sexual intercourse places a lot of stress on this area, and the potential for injury is great. These squamous cells are well used to handling threats from the outside world.

Where the squamous epithelium of the vagina and ectocervix meets the columnar mucosa of the endocervix is called the *transformation zone,* or *T zone.* This is the most vulnerable area of the cervix. Allow me to explain. The transformation zone begins its life as the more unglamorous sounding *squamocolumnar junction,* from the beginning of a girl's life until puberty. The squamocolumnar junction is, as the name implies, where the squamous and columnar epithelia join (see Figure 2.3), and is located on the outer surface of the cervix just beyond the os. (See Figure 2.4A.)

When a girl goes through puberty, her uterus and cervix enlarge significantly, which has a balloon-like effect on the mucosa of the cervix. That is, the enlargement actually stretches and pulls the original squamocolumnar junction toward the outer edge of the ecto-cervix. As a result, the central portion of the cervix around the os is covered by glandular mucosa. (See Figure 2.4B.)

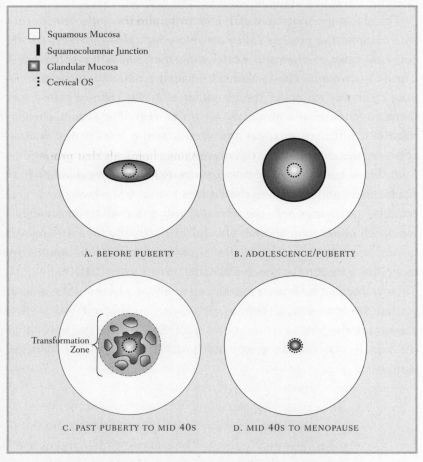

FIGURE 2.4 A GYNECOLOGIST'S VIEW OF YOUR CERVIX AT FOUR PHASES IN LIFE

So the adolescent now has a problem (among so many other problems that adolescents have). Remember that squamous epithelium is very good at protecting surfaces from the outside world. Now the adolescent's ectocervix is partially covered with glandular epithelium, which is relatively susceptible to injuries. Over the ensuing years, the body solves this problem by slowly re-covering this portion of the cervix with squamous epithelium. Hence, the name, transformation zone—in this area, the epithelium transforms from glandular to squamous. (See Figure 2.4C.) As we will see later, this has profound implications in terms of the development of disease.

This transformation from glandular to squamous epithelium occurs by a complicated process called *squamous metaplasia,* which actually consists of two mechanisms working together. The first mechanism is a brute force approach in which the original squamous epithelial cells nose their way up under the glandular cells, lift them off the basement membrane, and physically push them off. The second mechanism is a bit more mystical and occurs at the level of the reserve cells—remember, they are the dividing cells of the glandular epithelium. These reserve cells decide that this environment is way too hostile for them and reprogram themselves so that when they divide and produce a daughter cell, the new cell will differentiate into a squamous cell rather than another glandular cell. By the time a woman is in her late thirties or forties, the squamocolumnar junction slowly moves back into the endocervical canal. (See Figure 2.4D.)

Now that you have been introduced to all the players in the drama, you are ready to watch them in action—to understand how a virus can invade the female reproductive tract, how cancer can develop in the female reproductive tract, and how HPV in particular does its damage.

3

How Can a Virus Cause Cancer?

We all know the two basic words "virus" and "cancer." We generally regard the first as a nuisance (unless we're talking about AIDS, when we react with fear) and the second as a life-threatening menace. But few of us really understand what a virus actually is, what cancer actually is, and how the two might be linked. This chapter will teach you about viruses and about cancer. In the next chapter, we'll home in on HPV and look at how it causes cervical cancer, as well as other conditions.

THE VIRUS: DNA WITH A MISSION

A virus is the smallest form of life we know, and the ultimate parasite. All viruses consist of little more than a package of genetic material—

DNA or the less well-known molecule RNA—and a covering that allows the virus to attach itself to a cell and shoot that genetic material into the cell. The virus, like most forms of life, has a single mission: to reproduce itself. This is its sole purpose and its entire extremely efficient design has evolved to let the infected cell do all the work of reproduction. Having entered the cell, the virus uses the cell's own internal machinery to reproduce the viral genetic material and to make the proteins required to package the genetic material. Once this is done, millions of new viruses bud from the cell membrane to head out and infect other cells. Unlike the more complex bacteria, which divide and reproduce using their own machinery, the ingeniously designed virus uses your body's own machinery to accomplish its end. Thus, it turns the cells of your body into nothing more than a virus factory.

VIRAL REPRODUCTION METHODS

While reproduction is the mission of every virus, all viruses don't go about this task in the same way. Viruses differ in the time and method they use to accomplish their goal. When a virus wants to take over your cells, it can set up several possible "arrangements" with the host cell. We know most of the arrangements viruses can set up with cells, although we don't always know the details of how and why one particular arrangement is chosen over another. Understanding these possible deals that the virus can set up with the infected cell is important because it helps us understand how viruses are transmitted and why different people are affected in different ways by the same virus. It also helps us understand why some of these deals are more likely to cause a cell to go haywire and become cancerous.

Latency
The first arrangement is the "hang-around-and-don't-cause-any-trouble-for-a-while" approach. In this situation, the virus's genetic material enters the cell and basically does nothing. It just sits there and enjoys

the warmth and comfort of the host cell. This arrangement is called *latency*.

Productive Infection

Another arrangement is the enlightened self-interest approach. The virus realizes it has a pretty good deal, but it still needs to reproduce. So it uses the cell's own machinery to convert the cell into a virus factory, but it doesn't interfere with the cell enough to kill it. This arrangement is called a *productive infection* and is often the situation when a person is a carrier of a virus without actually showing any symptoms. As we'll see, viruses that cause productive infection are a rather insidious group of viruses because they can infect others without the person ever suspecting that he or she is a carrier.

Productive Infection with Cytopathic Effect

A yet more aggressive deal is a productive infection in which the virus ultimately kills the host cell. This is called *productive infection with cytopathic effect*. The virus figures, "So what if I kill this cell? By the time I do, millions of new baby viruses will have infected healthy cells around this one, and they can each decide what kind of deal they want to set up with their host cell. I have accomplished my mission and can rest happy." I call this the "kill-the-host-spread-the-word" type of infection.

Integration

The most sneaky and, as you will see, dangerous deal that a virus can enter into with the cell is to use it as a hideout. When a virus realizes that the body's immune system has gotten wind of its presence, it needs to hide in order to survive. It has worked out a slick and sinister plan to do this. A virus in a cell is not much more that a small piece of DNA floating around in the cell. What better location for a little piece of DNA to hide than in a big piece of DNA? And there are lots of big pieces of DNA, called chromosomes, in the nucleus of every cell in your body. But even worse, the viral DNA doesn't content itself with just floating around independently and hiding between your chromosomes. Instead, it actually splices itself right into your own chromosomal DNA so that it's next to impossible to find. This is called *integration*.

The amazing and dangerous thing about a virus is that after it infects you, it can try out these various deals when it sees fit. Some viruses go through cycles of nonproductive and productive infection. A well-known example of this is the herpes simplex virus. Genital and oral herpes cause painful sores that fester for a while and then heal. The sores are caused by the third "deal"—a productive infection with cytopathic effect. Your dying host cells contribute to the formation of the sore. Needless to say, all that activity doesn't go unnoticed by your immune system, which charges into the area, guns blazing, and decides that the only way to stop this process is to start killing everything in sight—specifically the viral-infected cells. This adds to sore formation. So now there's outright war, and the virus is panicked. What to do? Where to go? But the herpes virus isn't stupid. When the heat gets too strong, it just shuts down its activity and either becomes latent or goes into hiding and integrates into your cellular DNA, until the immune system thinks there's no more action and focuses on another area of bodily infection.

But your immune system isn't stupid either. It's always on the alert for the reappearance of the virus. As soon as it detects reappearance, it sends in the troops. And that generally keeps the body free of recurrence. But when you are stressed or when you are not living a healthy lifestyle, your immune system malfunctions. It will take its eyes off the hidden herpes bug long enough for the virus to start up its productive infection again. Lo and behold, you've come down with those nasty lesions again. The particular circumstances that trip up your immune system are often as unique and individual as you are. Most people with recurrent herpes know what is likely to cause an outbreak of lesions. Often it is times of stress, or advancing age, when the immune system, like the rest of the body, is not as strong as it used to be.

Now that you have been introduced to viruses, we can turn our attention to the other side of the story—cancer.

CANCER: DNA THAT'S RUN AMOK

What is cancer? Where does this disease come from and how does it start? While scientists are still hard at work unraveling the complicated set of knotty questions, some of the strands have become clear and a great deal is known. The story of cancer begins in the nucleus of the cell, where the DNA resides.

Before we can understand cancer, we must discuss DNA, which is another household word. Most people know that DNA is the building block material of genes. But few people understand exactly what it is or how it works.

The discovery that genetic material is made out of DNA began the modern era of biologic research. DNA, which is short for *deoxyribonucleic acid,* is often described as the blueprint for all cells. A better analogy sees it as the central microprocessing unit in your computer. Nothing happens within the cell without its direction. The instructions present in DNA are responsible for all cellular structure and function. DNA directs whether a cell is a stomach, muscle, or skin cell. If it's a skin cell, the DNA determines whether the skin is pale or dark. Everything a cell is and ultimately all that we are is coded in this long, thin, coiled molecule that is stuffed inside the nucleus of almost every cell in your body. DNA doesn't actually do the work. Rather, it directs the formation of proteins that carry out its instructions. But make no mistake, DNA is in charge, and if the DNA is damaged in any way, or if its instructions are not carried out correctly, the consequences for a cell can be death.

In the last chapter, we looked at the process of cellular renewal and maturation and death. It should come as no surprise that this process occurs under the direction of DNA. This is a very complicated and tightly orchestrated procedure. One protein causes a cell to divide, others tell the cell to stop dividing and start doing its job, and yet other proteins cause the cell to die.

All cancers are caused by this malfunctioning of the cellular DNA. In this book, however, we are concerned especially with cancers of the epithelium, or *carcinomas* (rather than with, say, sarcomas, which arise in bone and muscle, or leukemias and lymphomas, which arise in the blood system). The remainder of this chapter will focus on epithelial cancer and, in particular, how the cancerous process unfolds in the squamous and glandular mucosa of the cervix.

The basal cells on the basement membrane that do all of the dividing have a lot of growth proteins—their "accelerator" is switched on, if you will. The maturing cells in the middle of the epithelium have the cellular "brakes" on, and most of their time is spent organizing the proteins they need to become good protective squamous cells. Finally, the cells at the top—the ones that are dying, sloughing off, and being constantly replaced—have a lot of "death proteins." It's their job to self-destruct, because their work has been done: they're old, and it's time for new cells to take over. If you look back at Figure 2.3 in Chapter 2, you will see what the cells look like at various stages of maturation.

Cancer is a disease in which the orderly process of cellular birth, maturation, differentiation, and death has gone haywire. The result is that cells multiply uncontrollably and forget about what their job was in the first place. This uncontrolled multiplication can occur by malfunctions in one, two, or all three aspects of the cell's normal life cycle: increase in the growth rate of the cells—that is, the accelerator becomes permanently floored; a loss of the cell's brakes; and a malfunction of the self-destruct button. The result is cancer—a car with no brakes and a floored accelerator careening down a winding road right toward a crowd of people, with no self-destruct button to hit.

Even though this picture I have painted of cancer development seems like a wild haphazard ride toward destruction, the development of cancer does go through some recognizable phases. It appears that most cancers develop from a single cell in which all three mechanisms—those responsible for growth, growth-arrest, and self-destruct—have been compromised. This cell divides uncontrollably, soon giving rise to a whole population of equally damaged "cars" going down the mountain without brakes. This original cancer cell and all the cells that arise from it are called *clones*.

In cancers that develop from epithelial cells, this uncontrolled division of clones initially starts to replace all of the normal cells next to it on the basement membrane. Just like a invading army, these dividing cells push aside the normal cells because they are growing so fast. The new cells begin to pile up on top of one another.

Needless to say, if you look through the microscope at this phase of cancer development, you will not see the very ordered population of dividing cells at the bottom and functional cells in the middle and dying cells at the top. Instead, you'll see a microscopic free-for-all with a bunch of cells that are doing nothing but dividing, not trying to become protective squamous cells or secreting glandular cells, and all of them crawling on top of one another all the way up to the upper epithelial layers.

Initially, *all* of this mayhem takes place above the basement membrane. The destructive process, in other words, has not yet penetrated the basement membrane and entered the system. It's still highly localized. This precancerous stage goes by many names, including *dysplasia, precancer, noninvasive cancer, carcinoma in situ* (Latin for "cancer in its place"), and *intraepithelial lesion*. I might use these terms interchangeably, as might your doctor.

So what is the next step in cancer development? Cancers that arise in the epithelial cells—*carcinomas*—usually spend some time as wildly dividing clones sitting on the basement membrane, but the time frame for this stage varies from cancer to cancer. Eventually, unless it is removed by the surgeon's knife, a significant percentage of these carcinomas in situ get "fed up" with crawling along the basement membrane, and pull a cellular version of the Great Escape.

They start to tunnel out. When this happens, a group of rogue cancer cells (called *subclones*) somehow acquire the ability to cross the basement membrane and start growing down below the mucosa, into the submucosa. From there, they gain access to the blood and lymphatic vessels, which are the superhighways to the rest of the body. Once these cells have crossed the basement membrane, the whole process becomes an *invasive cancer.*

When the invasive cancer reaches a "superhighway"—a blood or lymph vessel—and decides to enter it for a quick ride, it now has the ability to *metastasize* or spread far away from the site of origin. This invasive cancer is what doctors are usually referring to when they say, "You have cancer." In fact, it is this invasion-and-spread that the physicians of antiquity had in mind when they chose the name "cancer" to refer to this particular disease process: Cancer is Greek for crab (the zodiac sign of cancer is represented by a crab). The invasive cancer acts, and under the microscope often looks, like a crab digging its way down through tissues with ragged claws.

What is the sinister force that makes good cells go so bad? The common theme in almost all cancers is some form of DNA damage. DNA, for all its wonderful talents, is a delicate molecule, and there are a lot of things in the hostile world that can hurt it. Radiation and toxic chemicals are good examples. We who live in the age following Chernobyl and toxic waste dumps such as Love Canal are all too familiar with how these exposures can cause cancers. Some people are also born with fragile or defective DNA, which make the cells more vulnerable to cancerous processes. The wear and tear of life itself can take a big toll on DNA. After all, every time a cell divides, the huge strands of DNA with its particular code must be copied exactly, without errors, and passed on to another cell. Your cells have an amazing mechanism to ensure that DNA is copied accurately. It resembles the spell-checking function in your favorite word-processing software. But even the spell checker can make mistakes, and our spell checker seems to become more fallible as we get older. The consequence is that an incorrect copy of healthy DNA, or a correct copy of damaged

DNA, is then passed on to all the daughter cells, like one bad photo-copy that's replicated over and over again.

Fortunately, those death genes and proteins that we talked about earlier can help us out in many of these situations. The process of cellular self-destruction is called *apoptosis,* which is Greek for "the falling of leaves from a tree." This is an illustrative image because it explains how controlled death is a part of the life process. These apoptosis genes and proteins are not only important in the natural death process in normal epithelium, but also are activated in times of dire cellular crisis—particularly when the cell's DNA is irreparably damaged. The importance of these apoptosis genes in the protection against the development of cancers is well illustrated by their name—*tumor suppressor genes.*

There is one more component in this process that works in our favor—the brave and loyal soldier cells of our immune system that patrol our borders and vanquish invading enemies. When the immune system is working properly, it can detect foreign infectious invaders and destroy them. Scientists today know that the immune system also has some ability to detect and destroy cancer cells. If your immune system has been weakened by other illnesses, damaging habits (such as smoking), poor nutrition, stress, or other unhealthful aspects of your lifestyle, it will be less effective in vanquishing invaders of all sorts—including cancer.

So How Are Viruses and Cancers Related?

As we said above, the common theme in the development of almost all cancers is DNA damage. We now know that viruses, like radiation and toxic chemicals, are also notorious DNA damagers. Remember that one of a virus's survival mechanisms is its ability to integrate itself into the host cell's DNA. It runs and hides wherever it can. There are many places in the extremely long molecular chain of DNA that a virus can squeeze into with no consequence at all to the cell. But there are other places where a hidden virus can be extremely destructive.

Let's say a virus hooks on to the gene responsible for encouraging cell growth and division—an "accelerator gene," to use our earlier analogy. If this virus happens to weasel itself into the particular portion of the gene that is the on/off switch, then the gene will permanently remain switched on. That causes the "accelerator" switch to remain on. The cell keeps dividing and dividing. The virus can similarly affect one of the "braking" or stop-dividing genes, turning it permanently off. The result is the same—the cell keeps dividing and dividing.

Here's a final nasty little trick that viruses pull. Rather than directly damaging DNA, many of them will force the cell to make a viral protein that has the specific function of inactivating the tumor suppressor (apoptosis) gene proteins. This will inactivate the self-destruct mechanism of a cell. It is pretty obvious why viruses have evolved this little mechanism—because it forces the infected cell to stay alive and become a virus factory, like a microscopic version of *Invasion of the Body Snatchers*. Of all the possible damage that viruses can inflict, this inactivation of apoptosis genes may be the most dangerous. A cell that can't die and is also infected with a DNA-damaging agent like a virus is the body's ultimate nightmare. This scenario increases the chances that one of the growth-control (accelerator) or stop-dividing (brake) genes will malfunction. Now the cell is on a dividing spree, and there is no way to stop it.

So am I saying that *all* viruses can cause cancer? That if you catch a cold, you should run to an oncologist? Emphatically not! Most viruses that we contract—the common cold, measles, stomach viruses, or chickenpox, for example—are not associated with the development of cancer. They seem to lack the ability to integrate into DNA and to inactivate the apoptosis genes.

How about HPV? Will this virus cause cancer? Sometimes, though not necessarily. It depends on many factors, including the particular strain of virus with which you are infected. The strains of HPV that are most likely to cause cancer are those that are best at inactivating the apoptosis proteins *and* that have a particularly good ability to integrate into human DNA. It also depends on the strength of your immune system and various lifestyle factors. The next chapter will look specifically at HPV—how it infects the female reproductive tract, what happens next, and how areas infected by the virus might develop into cervical cancer.

4

If I Have HPV, Will I Get Cancer?

At the end of the last chapter we said that infection with HPV *can* lead to cancer, but will not necessarily do so. Your next burning question is obvious: If I am infected with HPV, what are my chances of developing cancer, and what can I do to prevent it? This chapter will take you through various scenarios of HPV infection, including the progression from HPV to cancer. It will end with some suggestions for reducing your risk of developing cancer. We will return to those suggestions at much greater length in Chapter 11.

HPV TRANSMISSION

As mentioned in Chapter 2, the human papillomaviruses infect primarily the squamous epithelial cells of the body, including those covering the skin, mouth, esophagus, upper airways, urethra, anus, vagina, and ectocervix.

As you have learned, squamous cells are, by their very nature, highly exposed and accessible. Moreover, they're constantly being shed and replaced by new cells, as are all living cells on body surfaces. Understanding these two facts helps the virus's nasty little plot become clearer. The virus latches on to exposed squamous cells with appropriate receptors. Now we have an infected area. Despite the infection, however, the cells carry on their normal process of replication, cell death, and the shedding of the dead cells. In an infected area, the surface squamous cells that are sloughed off are actually the agents of transmission. Scientists do not know how long the virus can continue to live in a dead cell, but we do know that HPV is extremely hardy and can survive for some time outside the body of a living host.

If you could enlarge an infected squamous cell, you would see that it is covered with a fine layer of millions of new human papillomaviruses. In order to infect someone else or another location of your body, this cell ideally needs to sink into the deep layers of squamous epithelium, down near the basal cells—the ones that are doing all the dividing. This is actually not a hard feat to accomplish. Although your squamous epithelium is a tough suit of armor, it is subject to microbreaks or splits in the upper layers. These are not deep tears that are likely to draw blood, simply small splits. We all have dozens of these little splits. As I drag my arm across the desk, I probably incurred a few of these microtears. They're not painful and they probably heal or reseal moments after they happen, but they do expose the lower layers of the epithelium for a time. And if there is an infected squamous cell hanging around, it might get jammed down into one of these breaks, becoming a source of infection.

Microtears can occur as a result of any friction between the skin and some other surface, but especially during vigorous activities, such as sex. Sex creates a series of microtraumas, which can cause microbreaks. These offer the partner's HPV-infected squamous cells many portals of entry—particularly in the cervix, which is especially susceptible.

Now that you know how HPV is communicated, you can understand why it is one of the most difficult viruses to contain. Preventing its contagion is even harder than preventing contagion with HIV! During sex, there is a far greater exchange of skin cells than of body fluids, and the skin exchange is much harder to contain. Semen can at least be contained within a condom. But infected skin at the base of the penis and the scrotum are not covered by the condom. An infected man can easily pass the virus on to his partner. The reverse is also true, by the way. A man wearing a condom is protected from the fluids secreted by his partner during sex. But the exposed areas we mentioned above are not protected from her skin. Moreover, while HPV transmission directly into the vagina or cervix may be interrupted by condom usage, if passed to the external genital area, it can later be transferred into the vagina or cervix by something as simple as insertion of a finger, spermicide applicator, or tampon. The infected squamous cells can hitch a ride higher into the genital tract and infect these areas.

Another problem with HPV is that it's an extremely tough virus. Comparatively, the AIDS virus is pretty wimpy. It doesn't survive long outside of the body and is easily killed by a number of agents, including some spermicides used in condoms or other barrier methods of contraception. HPV, on the other hand, can survive for a long time outside the body—we do not know exactly how long.

Dead HPV-laden cells pose a risk of contagion to nongenital epithelial areas of the body as well. As you will learn in later chapters, one method of treating extensive genital warts is laser removal. During this procedure, surgeons and operating room staff must wear a special ultra-filter mask because even in the vapor that is generated from the lasered warts, infective viruses can survive and enter the nasal passages and upper respiratory tracts. They can take up residence in the nose, mouth, throat, and respiratory tract, causing warty lesions in these areas too.

WHAT HAPPENS AFTER HPV INFECTION?

Now that we know how HPV invades a cell, what happens after successful infection? Does a wart always develop at that site? Or if a woman is infected with one of the high-risk types, will she inevitably develop a precancerous lesion and then an invasive cancer? The answer to both questions is no. The story of what happens after HPV infection is much more complicated than this and not completely understood by scientists and doctors. Here's what we do know and understand. When a site in your body is infected by HPV, there are several possible outcomes. These outcomes are discussed below.

NOTHING HAPPENS

Obviously, this is the best scenario. Although the virus successfully invades the basal cells, the immune system immediately swings into action, attacking and killing the infected cells—and thus the virus. All the fanfare takes place on a cellular level. The infected individual doesn't even know that this battle has been fought and won because eradication occurs before any visible lesion appears. This outcome is highly dependent on several factors, including the number of tricks the virus has up its sleeve, as well as the integrity of the immune system, whether or not the immune system has been exposed to a particular viral type before. If the immune system has already been exposed, it may be primed to fight the particular strain of virus and may vanquish it quite easily. This is the principle behind vaccination—inject a tiny quantity of the organism into the body, and the immune system will have its battle gear in place so that if a person is exposed to a full-fledged quantity of the virus in the real world, the immune system is all set to go.

LOW-GRADE SQUAMOUS INTRAEPITHELIAL LESIONS (LGSIL)

A second possible outcome is a productive viral infection. The viral DNA directs all the cellular machinery to make new viral particles. The cells continue to reproduce at a slightly faster, though not uncontrolled, rate. This slight increase in cellular division creates more cells, and thus a wart can form. The newly born cells all contain the virus. This is probably the best deal for the virus. It gets to reproduce without endangering itself or its host. It can sit back and be satisfied.

A significant percentage of such infections do not form the classic raised skin lesion we know as a wart. These so-called flat warts are actually impossible to see without application of special solutions and the use of a good old magnifying glass. Both raised and flat lesions can occur not only on the external genitalia, but also internally—on the cervix, the vagina, and in the penile urethra of men. We will discuss this in greater detail in Chapters 7 and 9.

When this process affects the cervix, it is termed a *low-grade squamous intraepithelial lesion* (LGSIL). LGSILs are also known by doctors as *HPV cytopathic effect, koilocytic atypia, flat condyloma, mild dysplasia,* and *cervical intraepithelial neoplasia I (CIN I)*. The names *condyloma* and *condyloma acuminatum* may also be used; these refer specifically to the classic raised genital wart. The other terms are being replaced by the all-embracing "LGSIL" because our current understanding of this type of lesion is that it is low-grade, with a low probability of developing into cancer.

HIGH-GRADE SQUAMOUS INTRAEPITHELIAL LESION (HGSIL)

This is the worst scenario for both the virus and the host. The viral DNA integrates into the cell's own DNA, causing damage. The virus also inactivates the cell's tumor suppressor genes. Remember what we explained in the previous chapter: the cell's DNA contains a self-destruct mechanism in case the cell has become diseased. This protects the body from being overrun by a series of damaged cells. When the tumor suppressor genes are inactivated, the diseased cell can't self-destruct. The result is that very little viral replication occurs, which is, for the moment, bad for the virus. In fact, the only good thing about this situation for the virus is it gets to hide in your DNA. For the cell, however, this is a disaster. The inactivation of the tumor suppressor genes and the integration of the viral DNA into the host cells have the combined effect of promoting uncontrolled cellular growth and no self-destruct mechanism for these cells. This is called a *high-grade squamous intraepithelial lesion* (HGSIL), which is, in effect, a precancerous lesion. Left untreated, a significant percentage of them will go on to become invasive cancers. Other terms used for these lesions include *moderate dysplasia, severe dysplasia, cervical intraepithelial neoplasia II (CIN II), cervical intraepithelial neoplasia III (CIN III)*, and *carcinoma in situ*.

HGSILs are usually flat. Rarely are they visible to the naked eye. It is often necessary to coat the body surface with a special solution and/or to use special equipment to detect them. Figure 4.1 will give you a visual sense of what normal squamous epithelium, LGSIL and HGSIL look like under the microscope.

When I look at HGSIL under the microscope, I see the characteristic features of HPV infection in the cells coupled with more worrisome changes. Organization and order are lost. There are cells way above the basement membrane that are still dividing, and the nuclei of their surface cells are extra large and misshapen. This is what happens when cells with damaged DNA are allowed to divide uncontrollably. They stop caring about becoming functional squamous cells and focus most of their machinery on dividing. As they continue to divide, they continue to acquire genetic damage, and ultimately many of them can switch on the genes that they need to cross the basement membrane and become an invasive cancer. Therefore, the goal of

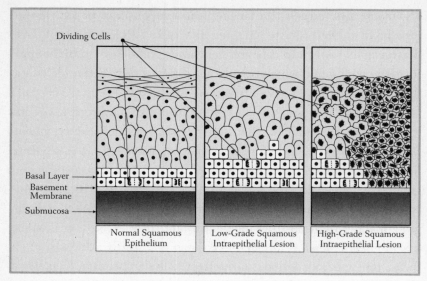

FIGURE 4.1 SQUAMOUS INTRAEPITHELIAL LESIONS

most screening efforts is to catch these high-grade lesions and remove them before they become invasive.

It would seem to follow that low-risk viruses cause low-grade lesions and high-risk viruses cause high-grade lesions, right? Wrong. At least once a week I have to dispel this concept from the mind of a fellow physician. Low-risk HPV almost always causes only low-grade squamous intraepithelial lesions (LGSIL), but high-risk HPV can cause either low-grade or high-grade squamous epithelial lesions (HGSIL). This is confusing, I know, but bear with me. Low-risk HPV strains rarely cause cancer because they cannot integrate into the cell's DNA or inactivate tumor suppressor genes. So they have to be content to merely take over cells and turn them into virus factories.

On the other hand, the high-risk viruses *do* have the ability to hide in your DNA, and they produce proteins that inactivate the cell's tumor suppressor mechanisms. But just because they *can* do this doesn't mean they always *will* do this. In fact, high-risk viruses are perfectly capable of setting up a productive viral infection—in other words, a low-grade lesion. In fact, the vast majority of LGSILs are caused by infection with high-risk HPV types. If high-risk HPV types were capable only of causing precancerous conditions without effectively making new baby viruses, then high-risk HPV would soon go the way of the dinosaur and become extinct.

So, where do these HGSILs come from? We really don't know. It is clear that some HGSILs do arise out of a LGSIL, but we are unsure about what makes a high-risk HPV that is causing a LGSIL decide to integrate into the DNA and set up the conditions necessary for a HGSIL to arise. It is also true that some high-risk HPV infections seem to rapidly decide to integrate and thus generate a HGSIL, apparently without ever causing a low-grade lesion. Again, what drives this is still a mystery. We do know that a key feature in the development of a high-grade lesion is how long the high-risk human papilloma virus is around before the immune system vanquishes it. The longer it takes for the immune system to get rid of the virus (a period referred to as *viral persistence*), the more likely it is to become a high-grade lesion. Viral persistence is affected by the ability of the immune system to contain the infection and also by the number of times a person is reinfected with high-risk HPV types. Again, key in determining viral persistence are the strength and effectiveness of the immune system and the presence or absence of such lifestyle factors as smoking and multiple sex partners. These determinants will be discussed extensively in later chapters.

ADENOCARCINOMA IN SITU (AIS)

Until now, our discussion has focused on what HPV does to the squamous epithelium. This is appropriate because about 90 percent of the cervical cancers lie within the squamous epithelium. However, genital HPV strains, usually high-risk types, also appear to have the ability to infect the glandular cells of the endocervix. This process is much more of a mystery to us. Indeed, it may not be a direct infection of the glandular cells, but actually may be an infection of the stem cells present at the cervical transformation zone that can become either squamous or glandular cells. When an infected cell divides and differentiates into a glandular cell, the result is an HPV-infected glandular cell with the ability to become precancerous and cancerous. A precancerous glandular process is called an *adenocarcinoma in situ*; a cancerous glandular process is called *invasive adenocarcinoma*.

Adenocarcinoma has been difficult to detect in the early stages until very recently, and its incidence is on the rise. Additionally, because it often brews in the endocervix, it is difficult to see even on close examination. Fortunately, we have some great new detection methods that are allowing us to find these lesions earlier. Indeed our ability to find these lesions at all may also be the reason that there seem to be more of them. These new detection methods will be discussed in Chapters 5 and 6.

THE NUMBERS GAME

The introduction stated that 60 to 80 percent of the American population is infected with HPV. But only a much smaller percentage of women develop LGSIL, HGSIL, AIS, and invasive cervical cancer— thank goodness! The question that is probably burning in *your* mind is the one we opened this chapter with: If I am infected with HPV, what are *my* chances of developing an intraepithelial lesion or cancer?

Let's start with the best news of all: current data indicate that about 90 percent of women infected with HPV develop no lesion at all—neither SIL nor cancer. How can that be? Remember the discussion about the various "what happens when a virus infects a cell" scenarios in the last chapter? It seems that the great majority of infections, whether from low-risk or high-risk strains of the virus, turn out to be latent: they infect the cell and "hang around and do nothing." It is also thought that many of the 90 percent of women who apparently don't develop an intraepithelial lesion really do develop some sort of lesion, but their superbly functioning immune system blows the lesion away so quickly that the screening doctors never have a chance to find it by their normal detection methods.

What if you are among the 10 percent of women who do develop a lesion that is detected? If you are infected with a low-risk HPV strain *only,* your chances of developing HGSIL, AIS, or invasive cancer is so small as to have some experts think it is zero. I don't like to say "never," so let's just say that your chances are very small. You can certainly develop a LGSIL, and indeed, there is data to show that approximately 10 percent of cases of LGSIL are caused exclusively by low-risk HPV infection. Several studies, again, show good news, specifically that the great majority (90 percent) of women will clear the virus down to levels undetectable by current methods within two years after infection; by three years after infection, nearly everyone has cleared the virus. It is very important to remember that this timeline assumes no reinfection with a different low-risk strain during that period.

Have I saved the bad news for last? Is the outcome different for women who develop an intraepithelial lesion as a result of infection by high-risk HPV types? The picture is much more complicated, but there is still considerable good news. The best study so far that systematically looked at what happened to a group of women infected with high-risk HPV *and* who developed a squamous intraepithelial lesion was done by a group of Dutch scientists and was published in 1999. It showed that after five years, 67 percent of these women cleared the HPV infection and the lesion. However, the other 33 percent did not clear the virus and had a persistent SIL. In many of these women the lesions progressed, that is they started out as LGSIL and became HGSIL. Clearly, this highly variable outcome in lesions caused by high-risk HPV reflects not only all of the possible virus-cell relationship scenarios, but also the ability of the person to get rid of the virus.

It is this group of women—the women with an intraepithelial lesion caused by infection with high-risk HPV who do not clear the virus—who are at the highest risk of developing an invasive cancer. This makes sense if you recall that HGSIL is really a cancer that has not yet acquired the ability to cross the basement membrane and become invasive. As much as 30 percent of these HGSILs may ultimately acquire this ability to invade. The problem is that as of now, we have no way of predicting which lesions will go away and which ones will become invasive cancer. Therefore all high-grade lesions are treated aggressively. If you have received such a diagnosis, you should not take it lightly.

The advent of Pap testing, discussed in the next chapter, has been extremely useful because it has flagged women with HGSIL and AIS. Identifying these women has enabled physicians to initiate treatment and most women who are correctly diagnosed and treated do not go on to develop invasive cervical cancer. Part of the reason why this has been such a successful screening and treatment method is that the time it takes for either HGSIL or AIS to become an invasive cancer seems to be relatively long. Although on a microlevel, the cells are proliferating at a frenzied and uncontrollable pace, on a macrolevel, the progression is actually slow. Remember that this slow progression does *not* mean you can wait around and neglect treatment of a lesion. Lesions can and do develop into invasive cancer and must be treated as soon as they are discovered.

WINNING THE NUMBERS GAME

In the previous section, you learned that most women who are infected with HPV do not necessarily go on to develop invasive cancer. So how can we predict who will develop cancer and who won't? Other than regular Pap screening and treatment, if warranted, what factors might be at play to protect these women against the disease? What risk factors make it less likely that these women will be protected and predispose them to the disease?

Scientists have identified several important risk factors. You will encounter some of them repeatedly throughout this book. As a pathologist who has performed biopsies on thousands of cancerous patients and who has seen firsthand the devastation that this disease brings, I become intense and passionate about bringing home the message of prevention. Many of the risk factors below can be avoided. That message cannot be repeated too often.

MULTIPLE SEX PARTNERS

It stands to reason that given the large number of HPV-infected adults in the United States, some if not all of your partners will be infected by the virus. It also stands to reason that given the large number of strains out there, some of your partners will be affected by one strain, while others may suffer from another. Obviously the more strains of virus you are exposed to, the more work you body has to do in order to fight them, and the more your immune system is overtaxed.

POOR NUTRITION

Chapters 10 and 11 will discuss nutrition in great detail, so I won't belabor the point here. I will say that adequate amounts of vitamins A, C, and E are known to have antioxidant properties, protecting DNA from damage. Some studies have linked folic acid deficiency with squamous intraepithelial lesions. Incorrect nutrition can contribute to a problematic balance between the two female hormones estrogen and progesterone. As you sill see in Chapter 10, this condition— known as *estrogen dominance*—has been linked with cervical disease.

Poor nutritional habits can cause many different types of cancer, not only cervical cancer. The American Cancer Society has issued nutritional guidelines advising people to lower fat intake and increase their intake of vegetables—especially the leafy green ones—and fresh fruits. These help protect against all forms of cancer.

PRESENCE OF OTHER SEXUALLY TRANSMITTED ORGANISMS

Interestingly enough, as scientists search for other missing pieces in the puzzle of cervical cancer development, some data suggest that infections with other organisms—particularly chlamydia—may promote the development of cancer in women infected with HPV. The mechanism is unclear, but it is thought to be a combined effect of the inflammation stimulated by another infection, which causes increased cellular division and an extra burden placed on your immune system at the site. It's easy to imagine how your immune system may be so preoccupied with fighting one invader that it may not be able to take on another invader.

SEX AT AN EARLY AGE

Remember our discussion of the cervical transformation zone? This is the area where cells "decide" whether to become squamous or glandular. As we explained in Chapter 2, this is a busy area of the cervix, and its constant state of activity makes it vulnerable. Sometimes there are more squamous cells, sometimes more glandular cells. Always, there are cells in the process of differentiating. It's as if they don't quite know their identity and are going through a struggle, rather than being solid, stable, mature citizens ready to withstand any onslaught. Cells in the transformation zone are more vulnerable.

The transformation zone of a young woman in early adolescence until her early twenties is larger and closer to the entrance of the vagina than that of a mature woman, as we discussed in Chapter 2. This vulnerable area is therefore more prominent and more exposed. Some researchers hypothesize that sexual activity during this sensitive early time makes it easier for HPV to cause infection for two reasons. One is that the transformation zone is simply bigger and more exposed, making it an easier target. The second reason is that the immune system of an adolescent is, like the rest of the adolescent, still growing. It may not be mature enough to effectively combat the virus.

Remember that the virus may not show up immediately. Just because a fourteen-year-old doesn't develop genital warts (although some do—I've seen them) doesn't mean she is free of the virus. It may have hidden in her DNA and may be latent. I have performed biopsies on tissues of young girls with LGSIL, HGSIL, and AIS. Recently, I had to advise the gynecologist treating an eighteen-year-old to proceed with a hysterectomy because the precancerous cells had spread too far into the endocervix to be removed any other way. While this is an extremely unusual scenario, the sad fact that it was unavoidable points to another sad fact: Sexual activity at a young age can have devastating consequences. After all, the only way a woman as young as eighteen could develop such an extensive precancerous lesion is by beginning sexual activity at a very early age.

SMOKING

This pernicious habit affects not only the lungs but also the whole body. While the lungs are the most obvious affected area because the smoke and nicotine actually enter them and swirl around in there, the effects are systemic. The harmful chemicals present in cigarette smoke are actually present in high concentrations in the cervical mucus of female smokers. These chemicals are believed to contribute to the development of cervical cancer in HPV-infected women by many different means, which include direct DNA damage to the cervical cells and a localized suppression of the immune system.

SUBSTANCE ABUSE

Alcohol weakens the liver. But even before the liver becomes seriously diseased, its functioning is significantly compromised by heavy drinking. As you will see in Chapter 10, the liver is a very important organ and is intimately involved in the processing of female hormones and the maintenance of a healthy female reproductive tract.

Drugs do damage in a variety of ways. Some directly attack DNA. Others weaken the immune system so that it is less effective in fighting off all infection, including HPV. An indirect result of drug and alcohol abuse is that when people are under the influence of these substances, their judgment is impaired. They are less likely to be discriminating about sexual partners and often find themselves in bed with a stranger, unsure of how they even got there. Being high or drunk can lead to promiscuity, which is a medical problem, not necessarily a moral one, as we discussed above. Of course, the ability to take proper precautions to protect against STDs is likewise compromised when under the influence of alcohol.

Eliminating these risk factors does not constitute an airtight *guarantee* that you won't develop cervical disease. But it certainly increases your chances of health greatly. Additionally, all of these factors contribute to other forms of cancer, not to mention heart disease and other health-related problems.

So how can you protect yourself against cervical cancer, beyond cutting down on the risk factors discussed above? The next chapter will discuss the Pap smear—a simple screening test that can detect cervical changes long before they become cancerous.

5

The Pap Smear—The World's Best Medical Test

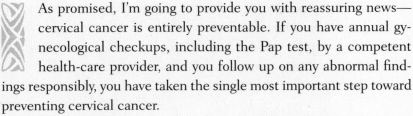 As promised, I'm going to provide you with reassuring news—cervical cancer is entirely preventable. If you have annual gynecological checkups, including the Pap test, by a competent health-care provider, and you follow up on any abnormal findings responsibly, you have taken the single most important step toward preventing cervical cancer.

This chapter will introduce you to the simple test that has been the most effective cancer-screening device in the history of medicine—the Pap smear.

What Is a Pap Smear?

The Pap smear, or Pap test, is short for *Papanicolaou test,* named after Dr. George Papanicolaou. This remarkable physician introduced his cell-sampling technique in 1949, and since then, it has reduced the incidence of cervical cancer in the United States by 75 percent over the past forty-five years. The Pap smear screens for premalignant changes of the cervix—in other words, the squamous and glandular intraepithelial lesions we discussed in Chapter 4.

As mentioned, the Pap smear is a *screening* test, not a diagnostic test. A diagnostic test is done to determine whether or not a person has a specific disorder. A screening is a first step in a diagnostic process. It is done to determine whether a given disorder might be present, and then sends those people who might be affected for further diagnostic work.

The purpose of a screening test is to survey a very large at-risk population and narrow down the individuals who may be suffering from the disease or condition being investigated. Once the screening test has highlighted people with a *possible* problem, diagnostic tests can determine whether an *actual* problem is there, and if so, what it is.

Why perform a screening to determine if you have a *possible* problem, when reliable diagnostic tests are available to determine whether you *definitely* have an actual problem? Screening tests provide an initial way of weeding out people who need further evaluation from a larger population. In other words, the goal of a screening test is to avoid subjecting a very large group of people to diagnostic tests, which can often be more invasive, uncomfortable, and expensive.

Other examples of screening tests include the standard hearing tests given to grade-school children and mammograms. The hearing test merely alerts the doctor to the presence of a possible problem. If a child does poorly on a hearing test, doctors must investigate further to determine just what the problem may be. Likewise, a mammogram is not a test for breast cancer, but rather a test that can alert the doctor to changes in breast tissue that *could* be a sign of cancer. If we didn't have mammograms, then every woman would have to undergo regular breast biopsies—an untenable option. Similarly, the Pap smear screens a large number of people at risk—the entire female population—and certain abnormalities detected on Pap smears will then require a true diagnostic test, a cervical biopsy.

Keep this distinction in mind as you go through this chapter. It will become especially important in the next chapter when we discuss how the Pap smear is interpreted and what you should do if your findings are abnormal.

A Pap smear is a routine part of the annual gynecological exam and is performed on women who show no signs or symptoms of cancer. Women who are showing possible signs of cancer will often be biopsied immediately rather than going through the screening procedure.

Although the primary focus of the Pap smear is the detection of squamous intraepithelial lesions, a considerable amount of secondary information can also be gained from looking at the cells of the cervix. For example, a woman's hormonal status can be determined by looking at cervical cells—the maturation of these cells is governed by the female hormones estrogen and progesterone. The relative balance of these hormones affects the microscopic appearance of cervical cells. Infections with other organisms such as herpes, chlamydia, and trichomonas can also be found with the Pap smear.

I consider the Pap test the mousetrap of diagnostic medicine because it is so effective, yet so simple in design. In fact, it's so simple, it's amazing that no one came up with it before 1949.

How does the Pap smear work? As we've discussed in previous chapters, the squamous and glandular epithelial surfaces of the vagina and cervix are always in a state of renewal. This benefits you because it keeps your cellular armor fresh and hence more effective. Unfortunately, viruses such as HPV have learned to exploit this process of renewal because they use the cells shed from the epithelial surface as the vectors, or agents, of infection. It makes sense, then, that one should be able to collect these cells that are naturally being shed all the time and see what they look like under the microscope. You may yourself have done this simple experiment in your high school biology class. You might have scraped your cheek and spread the cells onto a glass slide, then examined what they looked like under the microscope. This is exactly the principle of the Pap smear. We look for cellular abnormalities that point to the presence of HPV infection.

WHO SHOULD HAVE A PAP SMEAR?

The Pap smear is an essential part of good health maintenance for any woman over the age of eighteen, and for younger girls who are sexually active. Tests are generally performed every year.

There has been some controversy surrounding the question of whether a woman who has had a hysterectomy should continue to have annual Pap smears. My own opinion is that one should err on the side of caution. This is a relatively inexpensive and noninvasive test that can detect the presence of abnormalities in the region. Even after hysterectomy, a woman can be susceptible to cellular changes caused by HPV, and can go on to contract vaginal or vulvar cancer. And at any age and under any circumstances, a woman who is sexually active can contract HPV.

HOW IS A PAP SMEAR ADMINISTERED?

The Pap smear is a quick, painless procedure. It takes only a matter of minutes. Doctors and other specially trained health-care professionals, including nurse-midwives, nurse practitioners, and physician assistants, are qualified to administer it. Patients are most commonly tested in the doctor's office during the annual checkup, but can also be tested in a clinic or in an outpatient hospital facility. There is no need for hospitalization.

The woman lies on an examination table with her hips and knees bent and feet placed in stirrups at the end of the examination table. The doctor then carefully inserts a lubricated (and usually warmed) *speculum*—a metal or plastic device that spreads the vaginal walls, allowing the practitioner to see and gain easier access to the upper portion of the vagina and the cervix—to widen the opening. The doctor uses a miniature spatulalike instrument to scrape the surface of the ectocervix and endocervix right at the transformation zone. Usually a physician will also use a brushlike instrument inside the endocervical canal to ensure collection of the glandular cells. All of this can be felt by the patient, but, again, it is not painful. Immediately after collection, the cells are smeared onto a glass slide. The physician then uses one of many fixative solutions to preserve the specimen for transportation to the laboratory.

MAXIMIZING THE ACCURACY OF YOUR PAP TEST

While the Pap test is generally pretty accurate, there are some things that you can do to make it the most effective test possible. Here are a few tips:

- Honestly inform your health-care practitioner of your sexual history and current sexual practices and of any history of genital warts or other sexually transmitted disease.
- Do not douche for twenty-four hours before your Pap test.
- Try to schedule the test for a time when you are not menstruating.
- Do not use a tampon for twenty-four hours before the test.
- Do not use any vaginal medication—cream or suppository—for twenty-four hours prior to your test.

- Avoid sexual intercourse for twenty-four hours before your test. The semen itself, as well as any lubricant or spermicidal cream or jelly, can interfere with collection.

Some physicians believe that these precautions are not necessary for a routine Pap test. They believe that recent sexual activity, including use of lubricant or spermicide, or menstruation will not pose a problem. Speaking as a pathologist, I can tell you that any competent cytotechnologist should be able to distinguish between a blood cell, a mucus cell, residual lubricant, and a cervical cell. But sometimes there may be so much mucus, blood, or inflammatory cells that the "bad" cells can be obscured. So if you're having a follow-up or repeat test due to an initial problematic finding, you want to maximize accuracy as much as possible, and then these precautions become especially important. Of course, under all circumstances, you should inform your physician of any history of potential HPV-related conditions, and of your sexual history. And ask what you should do to prepare for your Pap test, since different physicians sometimes have different protocols and recommendations.

How Is the Pap Smear Processed and Examined?

When the preserved Pap smear slides are received at a laboratory, they are dipped into a series of staining solutions, called (of course) Papanicolaou stains. These stains make the cell nucleus and cytoplasm visible. The stained slide is then given to a *cytotechnologist*. In my opinion, cytotechnologists are among the great unsung heroes of medicine. They examine each slide, cell by cell, and identify cellular abnormalities, no matter how small. When they encounter an abnormality, they use a simple, old-fashioned technological device—an ink pen—to put a dot next to that questionable cell. After reviewing the entire slide, the cytotechnologist then judges whether any cellular abnormalities even remotely suggest the presence of a squamous intraepithelial lesion. If the answer is yes, the Pap smear is given to a trained pathologist, such as myself, to thoroughly review and make the final judgment regarding the nature of the cellular abnormality.

By law (as a result of the Clinical Laboratory Improvement Act discussed below), 10 percent of all Pap smears that a cytotechnologist deems as being "normal" must be reviewed by another cytotechnologist or pathologist. This practice helps provide quality control. Regulations also mandate that the cytotechnologists maintain records of the results of each random test and that they document all errors. Too many errors may result in loss of practice privileges—a highly stressful work situation indeed, as my own excellent staff of cytotechnologists will tell you.

THE CRISIS OF 1987

In 1987, many of *The Wall Street Journal*'s headlines were devoted to the great stock market crash in October. However, two articles also published in this revered paper concerned not an investment crisis but a medical crisis—the high "miss rate" of Pap smears. Of course, reportage of this medical crisis heralded financial catastrophe for many Pap smear laboratories and brought about a crisis in confidence in the Pap smear, the repercussions of which are still being felt today. The reporter Walt Bogdanich wrote these two articles, exposing the lack of uniform laboratory standards and the overworked conditions of cytotechnologists at many laboratories across the country. Unfortunately, these conditions had led to a number of errors, the most disastrous of which involved the failure of many cytotechnologists and pathologists to identify very small populations of premalignant cells. Many cases of cervical cancer were not detected and some of the affected women actually died as a result of these errors. It emerged that some cytotechnologists were required to look at more than 120 slides each day. Reading slides is exacting, finely detailed work, which requires alertness and complete concentration. Overworked cytotechnologists can easily miss a few tiny, stray problematic cells. Eyestrain, fatigue, and tedium take their toll. No human being can remain sufficiently alert and focused to flag a single cell with a slightly misshapen nucleus after looking at hundreds of slides containing literally thousands of cells.

The positive outcome of this article was a set of laws mandating and regulating the procedures of Pap smear laboratories. This set of laws, called the Clinical Laboratory Improvement Act (CLIA), was passed in 1988. Today's cytotechnologists are not allowed to review more than eighty slides a day, and their performance is subject to regular review. "Pap mills" have fortunately become a phenomenon of the past.

Despite the phenomenal improvement that the CLIA-88 regulations have brought to the practice of laboratories, the specter of poor performance continues to linger in the mind of the public. The famous British statesman Benjamin Disraeli once said, "There are three kinds of lies: lies, damned lies, and statistics." Certainly, this quote applies to some of the lingering distrust of the Pap test, because some distorted statistical spin makes the test look much more ineffective than it actually is.

LIES AND STATISTICS

What comes to mind when you read magazine headlines like "The Pap Smear Has a False Negative Rate of 25 to 30 Percent"? The vast majority of people, including both physicians and patients, erroneously think this means that 250 to 300 out of every 1,000 Pap tests are called "normal" when there is really a precancerous condition present. No wonder there is rampant fear—you certainly wouldn't board a plane on an airline with a "failure" record like that. But a *false negative rate* is a slightly more complicated calculation than its name would indicate. It is really a measure of the percentage of people who actually *have* the disease in which the test was inaccurate. For instance, take a group of 1,000 women. Let's say that 4 of them actually have cervical dysplasia. Now give all 1,000 women a Pap test, and let's say you find 3 of the 4 women with dysplasia—then you have a false negative rate of 25 percent. How? Well, you missed 1 of the 4 women with dysplasia and 1 of 4 is 25 percent. It doesn't matter that 999 of 1,000 women were correctly screened—the false negative rate is 25 percent because you missed 1 of 4 women with the disease. It most certainly does not mean that 250 of the 1,000 women have an inaccurate result.

While I do hope that this explanation exposes the negative spin often put on the Pap test with some fuzzy numbers—at the end of the day, it is still not much comfort to the one woman with the disease who was missed. And therein lies one of the inherent problems with the Pap tests—even the best mousetrap occasionally misses a mouse. For all its success as a medical test, the Pap smear is not perfect.

READING THE PAP TEST RESULTS

Now let's look at how Pap test abnormalities are classified. Like everything in medicine, terminology and classification evolve as increasing amounts of knowledge are accrued. The Pap test is no exception. Obviously, a test that has been around for more than fifty years has undergone numerous classification changes. However, the most significant advance occurred in 1993 with the creation of the *Bethesda Classification System,* which was revised in 2001. The system is still relatively young, so often Pap smear reports not only provide results with the Bethesda System but also provide results using older terminology.

While the entire Bethesda System is perhaps a bit too complex for discussion in a book of this type, let's discuss the most significant diagnostic categories, below.

REACTIVE CELLULAR CHANGES

This is a general category that includes all cellular abnormalities that a pathologist judges to be definitely unrelated to HPV infection and precancerous changes. Very often, a Pap test report will be a bit more specific about these changes. For instance it might read, "Reactive cellular changes secondary to candidiasis (yeast infection)."

LOW-GRADE SQUAMOUS INTRAEPITHELIAL LESION (LGSIL)

This category is used when squamous cells are present that show unequivocal evidence of infection by HPV. For most pathologists, these cells are easily recognized because they reflect the presence of a productive viral infection. What is not present is evidence of uncontrolled cellular growth and proliferation.

HIGH-GRADE SQUAMOUS INTRAEPITHELIAL LESION (HGSIL)

This diagnostic category is used when squamous cells that show unequivocal evidence of abnormal proliferation and lack of maturation are present. These features tell pathologists that a true precancerous condition exists.

ADENOCARCINOMA IN SITU (AIS)

This category refers to the same condition as HGSIL—with one crucial difference. The abnormal precancerous cells are not squamous but are glandular. Although the Bethesda System uses the term "in

situ," remember that we really don't know whether the cancer has re-
mained localized and "in its place" until we do a biopsy, which will tell
us whether the basement membrane has been penetrated.

CELLULAR CHANGES CONSISTENT WITH INVASIVE CANCER

This is an ominous diagnosis in which there are not only high-grade
intraepithelial lesion cells present, but also additional clues, such as
extensive bleeding and inflammation, suggesting that a true invasive
cancer has developed. This must be confirmed by biopsy.

ATYPICAL SQUAMOUS CELLS OF UNDETERMINED SIGNIFICANCE (ASCUS)

This is the most confusing diagnostic category and indeed has been
the most controversial category developed by the Bethesda System. It
is reserved for the vast "gray zone" of cellular changes that cannot be
conclusively attributed to one of the reactive changes and, by the
same token, cannot be conclusively attributed to HPV infection or
precancer. In an attempt to minimize this uncertainty, the original
Bethesda System divided ASCUS into various subcategories.

ASCUS without Qualification
This designation means that there are simply no other diagnostic
clues to help determine whether these cells are reactive, or HPV/
precancerous.

ASCUS Favor Intraepithelial Squamous Lesion
This subcategory means that atypical cells are present and lean more
toward the likelihood of HPV infection or a precancerous process.

ASCUS Favor Reactive Cellular Changes

This means that atypical cells are present and lean more toward the likelihood that a reactive process is taking place, based on a small number of other diagnostic clues.

Changes were made to this portion of the classification system in 2001. In the new system, ASCUS Favor Reactive Cellular Changes was eliminated, and ASCUS Favor Intraepithelial Squamous Lesion was retitled ASCUS Cannot Exclude High-Grade Squamous Intraepithelial Lesion. Your doctor may be still using the original terms, however.

ATYPICAL GLANDULAR CELLS OF UNDETERMINED SIGNIFICANCE (AGCUS)

This category is the same as ASCUS, except that the atypical cells in question are glandular rather than squamous. AGCUS also has a subcategory of Favor Adencarcinomi In Situ.

BUILDING A BETTER MOUSETRAP

Probably the most significant advance in screening for cervical disease since the original Pap smear was designed occurred in May 1996 when the Food and Drug Administration (FDA) approved new technology invented by a company called Cytyc. This new method is called *monolayer cytology testing*, which is more commonly known by its brand name, ThinPrep. The principle behind ThinPrep's improvement is as simple as the original Pap smear itself. Improvements begin at the level of collection and preservation. While the specimen is collected in the same manner—with a spatula and brush—the cells are not applied directly to a slide. Rather, all the collected cells are dipped into a solution, which immediately preserves the cells and breaks down any extraneous materials, such as mucus and many inflammatory and blood cells, which tend to obscure the cervical cells. The vial of preserved cells is then put into a sophisticated machine that evenly distributes the cells into a single layer onto a slide—hence the term "monolayer."

An esteemed fellow pathologist, Diane Solomon, M.D.—one of the authors of the Bethesda Classification System discussed previ-

DR. GEORGE PAPANICOLAOU

George Papanicolaou, M.D., Ph.D., was studying the hormonal maturation of the vagina when he discovered tumor cells in the vaginal fluid of women with cervical cancer. He presented his findings at a medical conference in 1928, but they were largely ignored. He did not give up, however. In 1941, he published a new paper on the subject, followed by his classic work, *Diagnosis of Uterine Cancer by the Vaginal Smear*, which was published with illustrations in 1943. The book focused on uterine cancer but also discussed the possibility of diagnosing early cervical cancer. The idea caught on and other gynecologists became enthusiastic about the possibility of finding an early intervention for cervical cancer and perhaps even eradicating the disease altogether. Actually, the first person to use the method that is known today as the Pap smear was a Canadian physician named J. Ernest Ayre. Rather than taking cells from vaginal secretions as Dr. Papanicolaou did, however, Dr. Ayre used a spatula to scrape cells directly from the cervix.

Laboratories performing these tests began opening in the 1940s, and by the 1950s, testing had become widespread. Despite all the computerized high-tech procedures of our age, this simple technique of a spatula and a glass slide has proved to be the single most effective tool in the prevention of any type of cancer.

In 1978, the United States government issued a commemorative stamp of Dr. Papanicolaou—a fitting but still small tribute to a man responsible for saving the lives of so many women.

ously—uses an excellent analogy to capture the nature of the mono-layer improvement. What would be the most effective way of visually locating the raisins in raisin bran? If you pour the cereal into a bowl, all you can see is the top layer. And just looking at the top layer, it's easy to miss the raisins because they can be hidden by the flakes. Certainly, raisins located underneath and at the bottom are completely invisible to the eyes. However, if you spread the cereal on a flat surface, it is not difficult to locate every raisin. Here, the "raisins" are the atypical cells and the "flakes" are the normal cells. Spread out in a single layer on a slide, it is much easier to identify which is which and to find the culprit cells.

ThinPrep technology also creates a clearer picture. Have you ever seen the smears left by muddy hands of children on your glass window? You really can't see out the window, much less detect bumps or the presence of grit in the smudgy mess. Here, too, a "smear" is less easy to work with than a clear background and by essentially "cleaning up the sample," cells become more visible.

Cytyc is not the only company trying to improve the Pap test. More recently, a company called TriPath Imaging has introduced a variation on the monolayer method called AutoCyte. Specifically, the variation employs a step designed to remove even more of the debris from the sample prior to putting it onto the slide. However, as of this writing, there has been no convincing clinical evidence that this method is superior to the conventional Pap smear in detection of low-grade and high-grade lesions. At this time, only Cytyc has received FDA approval to claim better rates of detection than the conventional method.

While the jury on TriPath's new Pap test technology is still out, TriPath has devoted considerable effort to the development and refinement of sophisticated computers that can screen Pap smears. Human eyes get tired, but computer "eyes" can keep going and never get fatigued. This technology, called Auto Pap, was born in the early 1990s and has been continuously developed since that time. Currently, TriPath has the only FDA-approved system for computerized mono-player Pap test screening. Despite phenomenal improvements in this technology and strong promise for its future, the method has still not gained widespread acceptance. This is probably because the technology is still very expensive and there are very few large-scale studies actually demonstrating that the computer is any better than a pair of well-trained and well-rested human eyes.

What Kind of Pap Test Should I Ask For?

Although the modifications to the Pap smear made by the ThinPrep method are now recognized as improvements over the conventional Pap smear, this new test was initially met with skepticism from the medical community. One of the major concerns was that "cleaning up" the sample may actually destroy the cancer cells in the first place. Over the past several years, however, numerous formal scientific studies from centers all over the world have confirmed that cells are not lost or destroyed in the process and that this method is significantly more effective than the conventional Pap smear in detecting both high-grade and low-grade squamous intraepithelial lesions and precancerous glandular lesions (adenocarcinoma in situ). Now medical skepticism is being rapidly replaced with widespread embracing of this test by gynecologists, pathologists, and patients. I think it is only a matter of time before monolayer cytology techniques are deemed "standard of care" in America. Currently, 51 percent of all women in the United States getting Pap tests are receiving a ThinPrep Pap test.

If you encounter resistance to ThinPrep testing on the part of your practitioner now, it's because he or she either may be unfamiliar with this new method or may be reluctant to change what he or she has been doing for so many years. Alternatively, this "well-meaning" doctor may be trying to save you money, since the ThinPrep method is more expensive. However, the typical cost difference between the conventional Pap test and the ThinPrep method is $25 to $35, and its use is covered by most insurance plans. For the price of two music CDs, you can have the added security of a better test, which may indeed save your life.

Now that you understand what Pap smears are designed to do and how they are processed and read, you're in a better position to know what to request. Ask your health-care provider for the newer mono-layer Pap technology. Insist on it, and don't let him or her tell you that it's not "standard of care." It should be *your* standard of care! The technology *is* available to reduce chances of a missed abnormality and increase accuracy, and you shouldn't settle for anything less.

Sometimes, well-meaning doctors may try to dissuade patients when they ask for this test to be performed. I know of several instances where patients asked for ThinPrep testing and were told that conventional testing is sufficient—despite what studies have shown. In this case, if your doctor will not honor your request, you should consider finding a doctor who will.

An acquaintance of mine—a lawyer, as a matter of fact—had been regularly receiving annual checkups and conventional Pap screening. When she read about the ThinPrep test in a magazine, she tried to convince her doctor to switch Pap testing methods. The doctor was reluctant at first, but she used the full weight of her formidable legal training to convince him to give her the newest technology. Lo and behold, when I looked at the Pap test, I found a high-grade lesion. Subsequent biopsy results showed very early invasive cancer. Fortunately, she was completely cured by hysterectomy. I shudder to think what would have happened had she not demanded this new testing.

In my own clinical practice, I have found that significantly more lesions are flagged by this new technology. Without exception, every gy-necologist I've worked with who has switched from conventional to ThinPrep testing methods has been shaken by the number of new cases of HGSIL and adenocarcinoma in situ being uncovered with this new method.

What You Should Know about the Lab That Reads Your Pap Smear

Fortunately, the CLIA-88 regulations have imposed a uniform set of standards on all American laboratories performing Pap tests. This has eliminated much variability in laboratories and has effectively eliminated the so-called "Pap mills" of the 1970s and early 1980s. However, there are some additional questions that you should ask your physician about the Pap smear laboratory he or she uses to ensure that you are getting the best possible care and the most accurate results.

IS THE LABORATORY CERTIFIED BY THE COLLEGE OF AMERICAN PATHOLOGISTS (CAP)?

The College of American Pathologists imposes even more stringent standards on laboratories and also requires laboratory personnel to take an ongoing series of tests to be sure they are interpreting slides accurately.

Make sure that the pathologist reading your Pap test is also certified by the American Board of Pathology in Anatomic Pathology. Some pathologists take an additional year of fellowship training in cytopathology and may have a subspecialty board certification. While all board-certified pathologists are qualified to interpret Pap tests, if you have any questions about your Pap results, you may request a second opinion from such a subspecialist in cytopathology.

WHY HAS YOUR DOCTOR CHOSEN A PARTICULAR LABORATORY?

The reassuring answer would be that the lab was selected based upon its record of accuracy of results, ease of interaction, and a rapid turn-around time. Beware if a physician has chosen a laboratory only because it's cheaper, or if the laboratory takes more than one to two weeks to provide the results.

DOES THE LABORATORY OFFER ADVANCED TECHNOLOGY SUCH AS THINPREP AND HPV TESTING?

These two tests represent unequivocal advances in cervical screening, and all good diagnostic laboratories should at least have these available. You will learn more about HPV testing in the next chapter.

WHAT IS THE LABORATORY'S POLICY REGARDING THE REPORTING OF RESULTS?

A good laboratory will personally notify your physician of a result of high-grade squamous intraepithelial lesion, adenocarcinoma in situ, or invasive carcionoma. Other laboratories directly notify patients by mail of normal results. Good communication between your doctor, your pathologist, and you is key!

DOES THE DOCTOR SEND THE PAP TESTS AND THE CERVICAL BIOPSIES TO THE SAME LABORATORY/ PATHOLOGIST?

One of the absolute necessities in the process of screening for cervical cancer is to correlate abnormal findings in a Pap test with the findings in the subsequent cervical biopsies or cone biopsies—if one is deemed necessary. If the specimens are being sent to different laboratories, then both laboratories are essentially operating in the dark, and you, the patient, are not getting the diagnostic service to which you are entitled. There is no good reason for the specimens to go to different labs.

WHAT CAN GO WRONG?

Despite the dramatic improvements in Pap testing discussed above, Pap tests are not foolproof. There are three major levels where the Pap smear can go wrong: collection, preservation, and screening. The first major error can occur at the point of sampling, or collection. A cervical lesion may be so small that it eludes the spatula or brush. These instruments either fail to capture the premalignant cells or may not effectively transfer the cells to the slide. Preservation is the next hurdle. The cells may be collected and may even be present on the slide but may not have been preserved rapidly or completely enough to be recognizable. Finally, at the screening level, the cytotechnologist or pathologist may simply miss a small population of atypical cells. The clinician may just overlook these cells due to fatigue or carelessness, but more often the problem is that the atypical cells "hide" behind other cells and are therefore not visible to even the most meticulous and observant set of eyes.

Historically, this imperfection has been accepted among physicians because we have long understood that cervical cancer is a relatively slowly progressing cancer so it usually takes a period of several years for a high-grade squamous intraepithelial lesion to progress to invasive malignancy. Unfortunately, no test is foolproof. The thought is that if we can get *every* woman to get a Pap test *every* year, then even if we miss the disease one year, we will likely not miss it the next year, and we will still have time to treat it. But increasingly, even this small error rate has become unacceptable to both physicians and patients, mainly because the consequences of even one miss can be the death of a woman from completely preventable disease. The desire to make this horrible outcome a thing of the past has driven several innovative companies to make some major improvements in this time-honored test.

The next chapter will examine one more improvement in Pap testing—the HPV test. It will also tell you what to do if your Pap test results are abnormal.

6

What to Do If You Have an Abnormal Pap Result

If you receive a disturbing result on your Pap smear, the most important advice is: Don't panic! Don't consume yourself with worry, and don't jump to the immediate conclusion that you have cervical cancer. By now, you should know that there are many categories of cervical abnormality, and they don't all lead to cancer. Even those that could become cancerous have now been detected and chances are that the progression of the disease can be arrested right now, before further damage is done. So once again, don't panic. *Do* review the last chapter to understand what your results mean and read this chapter to find out what the next step should be. Anxiety is a normal reaction, but this chapter will help allay some of your fears and will give you the information you need to make sensible, sound choices with your health-care provider.

Non–HPV-Related Reasons
for Abnormal Pap Test Results

The best-case scenario, of course, is that your Pap smear comes back normal. Although there are occasional false negative results, the technology we looked at earlier has significantly reduced this type of outcome, and you can breathe easy.

If your Pap smear has come back with an abnormality, don't panic! It doesn't necessarily mean that you have cervical cancer. Remember that it is a screening, not a diagnostic test. It can mean anything from nothing to "something strange" going on. The presence of abnormal cells can mean a variety of things.

To begin with, you might have some kind of infection, such as herpes or yeast. This can lead to an inflammation of the cervix, which is called *cervicitis*. Your doctor will probably repeat the Pap smear after you've been treated for the infection. Many physicians will choose to repeat a Pap test in six months after an abnormal finding that they attribute to cervicitis. This provides extra reassurance that the infection has not returned and, more important, that all the abnormalities were caused by the infection rather than by the cervical changes that herald the development of cervical cancer.

Atypical cells can be caused by a variety of other factors. Hormonal changes such as those accompanying pregnancy, miscarriage, or menopause can lead to unusual-looking cervical cells. Atypical cells can also be the side effect of medications such as Depo-Provera (a type of contraceptive), hormone replacement therapy (HRT), and certain drugs used in cancer chemotherapy. Interestingly, a severe deficiency in folic acid can also lead to strange cellular abnormalities because folic acid is an essential compound for your cells to make new DNA.

ATYPICAL SQUAMOUS INTRAEPITHELIAL LESION (ASCUS)

As we discussed in the previous chapter, ASCUS is a broad category indicating that "something strange" is going on, but we're not sure whether it reflects a reactive change due to another infection or hormonal fluctuation, or whether it reflects the presence of HPV and/or precancerous changes. Despite the fact that the creation of this category is completely logical, it has been, nonetheless, very frustrating for pathologists, clinicians, and patients alike. It is very difficult not knowing what's going on. I want to be able to provide a more definitive answer and say, "This is what you have." Your gynecologist would like to say, "I have results from the lab, you have such and such and here's what to do about it." Even better, "Your results are normal. See you next year." Instead he or she has to tell you that there *might* be a problem, but they're not sure what it is, or even that you definitely have a problem at all. And of course it's frustrating and worrisome for you, the patient. It's natural to wonder and even to spin out a series of worst-case scenarios. Although the subcategories of ASCUS are an attempt to clarify the situation, the end result of not really knowing what's going on is still the same.

The standard protocol following an ASCUS result has been two approaches:

- Wait three to six months, then repeat the Pap smear.
- Move on to the next diagnostic step immediately, which includes a colposcopy and/or a biopsy.

WAIT AND REPEAT

Watching, waiting, and repeating the Pap test is a conservative approach with both advantages and disadvantages. The advantages are clear. No inconvenience, no invasive procedures, simply a follow-up visit a few months later. If the problem has cleared up by itself, everyone feels relieved and the approach seems to be vindicated. The woman is not subjected to further uncomfortable and expensive procedures, and the problem has resolved without them.

But waiting has its downside too. The waiting period can be quite stressful for the patient. Studies have shown that the time of limbo following this confusing diagnosis exacts a psychological toll on women. And more often than not, a repeat Pap test will show the same "strange-looking" and inconclusive ASCUS cells.

So wait-and-repeat, like most other courses of action, has pluses as well as minuses. The decision to follow this course of action (or inaction) lies in the hands of your health-care provider.

COLPOSCOPY AND BIOPSY

Some doctors prefer to have all elements of uncertainty eliminated as soon as possible. They may opt to move on to the next step immediately by performing a *colposcopy*. Colposcopy is a relatively painless procedure in which a lighted microscope, called a colposcope, is used to view the cervix very closely, enabling your doctor to see the abnormal areas of the vagina and cervix that are not otherwise visible. The cervix is first stained with a vinegar or iodine solution, making any lesions more visible.

If a lesion is seen, the doctor will take a biopsy—the removal of a small piece of tissue from the affected area for analysis by a laboratory. Using the colposcope for guidance, the doctor will snip the tissue from the area with an instrument that somewhat resembles a hole puncher. Usually, the physician will also take an additional sample of the endocervix with an instrument called a *curette* that actually scrapes fragments of tissue out of the endocervical canal (this is called endocervical curettage). The biopsy specimens are placed on slides for examination by a pathologist. These biopsies show fragments of the entire epithelial surface, the basement membrane, and the submucosal tissue—a far more extensive sample than what's collected during a Pap test, which only examines the surface. In essence, we have a full thickness view of the entire area, and with the benefit of this view, the definitive diagnosis of the process is made.

As you can imagine, colposcopy and biopsy also have their downsides. The word "biopsy" sends chills of horror through most, who immediately conclude that they have cancer. Undergoing a biopsy can also be stressful and mildly painful. The procedure is slightly invasive and also costly. Fortunately, there appears to be hope on the way.

WINNING THE WAR ON ASCUS—HPV TESTING

While I said there "have been" only two standard protocols for ASCUS, the advent of a new test means that a third protocol is in the process of evolving and may well become standard practice in the coming years. A new test specifically to detect the presence of HPV has been approved by the FDA. This test has been developed by the company Digene and is called the Hybrid Capture II (HCII) test, but is usually known as the "HPV test." Very simply, it can determine the presence of a number of low-risk and high-risk viral types in a cervical specimen. Unlike the Pap test, it looks for the presence of viral DNA in the cells. The method used to do this is extremely sensitive and specific, and therefore very accurate.

The test utilizes the same cells remaining in the liquid-based collection of cells gathered during the ThinPrep Pap test we discussed in the last chapter. This means that the patient is not subjected to the stress of a new procedure to collect cells, with its inconvenience, cost, and accompanying worry about the possibly disturbing results of her original Pap test.

If the test is negative for HPV, it is strong evidence that the odd-looking cells are due to a reactive cause, such as hormonal changes or the presence of a different kind of infection. This information may lead your gynecologist to perform additional tests to help ascertain what else might be going on. But a negative HPV test does help provide a significant degree of comfort to both the patient and the physician that the cervical changes do not reflect a precancerous condition.

If the test is positive for the high-risk strains of HPV, then management is clear. In this situation, the presence of atypical cells plus the DNA of high-risk HPV presents sufficiently compelling evidence to warrant colposcopy and biopsy if a lesion is seen.

If the test is positive for only low-risk types of HPV, then the options are somewhat more controversial. There is a perfectly valid case for watching and waiting here: We can probably assume that the abnormal cells were caused by HPV infection, but since it's a low-risk type, the probability of its going on to cancer is extremely low, and therefore colposcopy and biopsy may be overkill. However, some physicians choose to couple all this information with their direct inspection of the cervix through colposcopy to reassure themselves and their patient.

There has even been some controversy as to whether testing for low-risk virus is useful. In my opinion, while low-risk virus has very little if any ability to become cervical cancer, coupling this testing with an ambiguous result like ASCUS often provides the patient and the clinician with some closure. They now know what's going on.

There is a further reason to have the HPV test done. It's more accurate and sensitive than a repeat Pap smear in detecting high-grade lesions. The ASCUS/LGSIL Triage Study (ALTS) is a major multicenter study that has been intensively looking at the role of HPV testing after an ASCUS or LGSIL finding. One of the many findings of this study is that HPV testing was more sensitive in detecting underlying high-grade lesions than was a repeat Pap smear in women with a previous ASCUS or LGSIL result.

Make no mistake: while the HPV test is extremely powerful, in my opinion and that of most physicians, the power of this test is only manifested when coupled with the Pap test. This leads to a logical question: If we have an effective test for HPV, and all cervical cancer is caused by HPV, why bother with a Pap test at all? Why don't we just test everyone for HPV? Good question. Here's the answer. Remember that studies show that between 60 and 80 percent of the population may be infected by HPV at some time in their lives. And remember the numbers game. Of this huge population, fortunately only a small percentage of people go on to develop precancerous changes. You can imagine that if you randomly tested people for HPV, you might expect a very large percentage of them to be positive, but without having developed squamous intraepithelial lesions—remember the various "arrangements" a virus can set up? Therefore, HPV testing is not an effective screening device because it doesn't do what a screening test should do—that is, narrow the group of people subjected to invasive diagnostic procedures. This is accomplished by the Pap test. The beauty of the HPV test is that it brings the sometimes ambiguous changes flagged by the Pap test into clearer focus. For this reason, I do *not* suggest that all readers put down this book and immediately run to their health-care providers, clamoring for an HPV test.

However, I urge readers with ASCUS to demand HPV testing. At the time of this writing, the HPV test is still relatively new, although the results of the ALTS trial are resulting in rapid acceptance. Many physicians are not yet aware of its existence and others feel it's un-necessary. In my own practice, I have become absolutely convinced that selective HPV testing, along with the monolayer Pap test, are two tools that could effectively eradicate cervical cancer in our lifetime. I am, therefore, very passionate in my promotion of both tests. My desire to effectively promote the value of these tests is without any self-interest. I have never accepted an honorarium of any sort from companies to provide physician education about these tests. I do not own a single share of stock in any of these corporations. I believe this would taint the message I so urgently want to impart, which is that the combination of the monolayer Pap test and the HPV test provides a simple and highly practical way to resolve a classic medical dilemma and provide solid answers that can save lives.

A personal story will illustrate the utility of HPV testing and why I feel so strongly about it. A patient of mine had received an ASCUS Pap test result sporadically over the course of several years. She mentioned this to a friend of hers, who happened to be a member of the secretarial staff at Digene, the manufacturer of the HPV test. Her friend urged her to have HPV testing, and after some pleading and foot-stamping, she managed to convince her gynecologist to order this "exotic" test. I looked at her Pap slide and, sure enough, I had to say "ASCUS." But when the HPV test came back positive for a high-risk strain of the virus, I advised her gynecologist to perform a colposcopy and biopsy. He did—and discovered a tiny high-grade lesion. It is likely that she would have continued showing ASCUS on and off for several years longer, while the lesion continued to grow. I believe that this test could possibly have saved her life.

ATYPICAL GLANDULAR CELLS OF UNDETERMINED SIGNIFICANCE (AGCUS)

Although in concept, the category of AGCUS is similar to ASCUS, the management options are often more problematic. As the name implies, AGCUS indicates that there is a population of atypical glandular cells and we're uncertain as to whether they reflect reactive, precancerous, or invasive cancerous changes. HPV testing can be of use but not nearly as much as in ASCUS. This is because atypical glandular cells may arise not only from the cervix but also from the endometrium, the fallopian tubes, and—uncommonly—even the ovaries. Remember that the entire female genital tract is a single connected pathway consisting of glandular cells above the transformation zone. So while HPV testing may help rule out the possibility of an endocervical adenocarcinoma, it does not help rule out cancers arising in higher structures such as the uterus, fallopian tubes, or ovaries. These processes do not necessarily result from HPV. Sometimes pathologists can be fairly certain that the atypical glandular cells are indeed from the endocervix. In this case, as you may predict, HPV testing may be very helpful. However, when this is not possible, it is very difficult to determine the origin of these abnormal glandular cells. Because of this, clinicians usually choose to more aggressively investigate the source of such cells by performing colposcopy and biopsy of the endocervix and even of the endometrium. Biopsy of the endometrium is taken with a small, strawlike instrument called a "pipelle."

Because of the complex management options involved with an AGCUS diagnosis, I would encourage an extensive dialogue with your health-care provider regarding the most appropriate management strategy for you. Unlike with ASCUS, the risks of a watch-and-wait approach are much higher here. If it were my wife, sister, or daughter, with an AGCUS, I would insist on at least an HPV test and probably the additional colposcopy and biopsy procedures.

Low-Grade Squamous Intraepithelial Lesion (LGSIL)

An LGSIL finding should always be followed by a colposcopy and biopsy. Biopsy is the definitive diagnostic procedure to determine what kind of lesion you have. If it confirms the presence of LGSIL, your doctor may take one of two approaches to the situation. In fact, LGSIL management is quite a controversial issue among physicians.

WATCH AND WAIT

Since most LGSIL lesions are unlikely to become precancerous or cancerous, it's reasonable to wait and see if the immune system kicks in and knocks out the lesion. As we mentioned in Chapter 4, most women with LGSIL do not go on to develop invasive cancer. Chances are good that the lesion will clear up by itself. Careful monitoring can ensure that the lesion doesn't spread or change in any way. This is a conservative approach that seeks to save women from possibly unnecessary surgical procedures and to preserve as much of the cervix as possible.

EXCISION OF THE LESION

This approach says, better not take any chances. A lesion is a lesion and should be removed. LGSIL lesions are usually caused by high-risk viral types. You never know when one of these high-risk strains decides to get nasty, go for the DNA, and cause a transformation to a high-grade lesion. The lesion is removed using the same procedure as the cone biopsy.

Current thinking leans toward the more conservative approach, and I am inclined in that direction myself—with a few caveats. It is crucial for your doctor to be absolutely certain that he or she can see the entire extent of the lesion. But the lesion may extend into the endocervical canal, enabling the lesion to "hide." In such cases, it's appropriate to excise the lesions, even if they're low grade, simply because you can't keep an eye on them (literally). "Watch and see" will only work if you can actually watch and see what's going on.

If your lesion is on the outside of the cervix, and your doctor can monitor what's going on, then it's reasonable to wait. In Chapter 10, Dr. Warshowsky will provide you with some tips that can enhance your immune system's ability to combat and, hopefully, vanquish the lesion during the period of waiting.

One little-discussed aspect of having a low-grade lesion: You are highly contagious. Remember that a low-grade lesion is a productive viral infection, which means that numerous new viral particles are always being made. During this period of watch-and-wait, be sure to inform your partner.

High-Grade Squamous Intraepithelial Lesion (HGSIL) and Adenocarcinoma in Situ (AIS)

When a biopsy confirms either of these diagnoses, regardless of their extent or location, you must have your lesion removed. This is because, as we discussed in earlier chapters, these lesions are true precancerous conditions. If left untreated, a significant percentage will not be eradicated by the immune system but will cross the basement membrane and become a life-threatening invasive cancer. We have no means of knowing which way a lesion will go and therefore we can't afford to take the chance.

There are two methods doctors use to remove lesions. Once the lesion is completely removed, it is sent to a pathologist to make sure there is no associated invasive cancer in the tissues that were not examined during the original biopsy and to make sure that the lesion has been completely removed.

COLD-KNIFE CONE EXCISION

In this procedure, which is generally done in a hospital setting under anesthesia, the physician cuts out the center of the cervix with a scalpel. It's like taking the core out of the center of an apple. The reason it's called a "cone" excision is that the tissue removed by the cervix is shaped like a cone. The scalpel is used to cut deep around the lesion so as to remove all of it.

Cold-knife cone excision is the first line treatment choice for AIS because of this lesion's propensity to extensively affect the endocervix, which is an area you cannot see. Therefore, the goal is to remove as much tissue as possible. However, many physicians have for some time believed that a cold-knife excision for HGSIL may be overtreatment and cause unnecessary damage and loss of cervical tissue. A major problem associated with this procedure is called *cervical incompetence:* so much muscle is removed from the cervix that the cervix is left unable to do what it's supposed to do—serve as a cuff to keep the uterus closed so that the fetus remains inside and germs remain outside. This can jeopardize a pregnancy.

LOOP ELECTROSURGICAL EXCISION PROCEDURE (LEEP)

In this procedure a local anesthetic is administered, and an electrified wire loop is used to cut through the cervix, removing the lesion and conserving much more cervical tissue and muscle. The wire cuts, burns, and cauterizes so it controls bleeding. LEEP has a much lower infection rate and much faster healing than cold-knife cone excision. It's currently considered the first-line treatment for cases of HGSIL. When the pathologist examines a LEEP specimen microscopically, it occasionally may be found that the high-grade lesion is so extensive that it was incompletely removed by the LEEP. In this case, physicians may choose to do a second LEEP, removing more of the cervix or to go directly to cold-knife cone excision.

WHAT YOU SHOULD EXPECT FROM COLD-KNIFE OR LEEP PROCEDURES

These methods of lesion excision are surgical procedures, and as such, may be scary. Let me address a few of your possible concerns below.

External Appearance
While there is always some concern about disfigurement and a change of body image following surgery, be assured that your external appearance will not be affected by either of these procedures.

Pain
Though little pain is experienced during the procedures due to the use of anesthetics, your physician will probably advise you to take some prescription or nonprescription medication afterward to control pain. You may experience mild pain, discomfort, and/or spotting afterward. You should not engage in sexual activity, use tampons, lift heavy objects, douche, or bathe for some period of time to be determined by your physician—usually at least a month.

Sexual Relations
Once the cervix has healed and your doctor approves, you may resume sexual relations—with the measures taken to prevent transmission of HPV, discussed in Chapter 9. There is no reason why this procedure should impede your ability to feel aroused or to achieve orgasm.

If you have any additional concerns, you might consider talking to your health-care provider or to a trained social worker or psychologist who has experience working with these issues. Other resources are listed in the back of the book.

NOW WHAT?

Once you've had the LEEP procedure done, your doctor will follow you carefully to make sure there is no recurrence of the lesion. Protocol is to have a follow-up colposcopy several months after LEEP, and then a Pap smear every four to six months until three consecutive Pap smears are normal. This is because lesions can recur, particularly if there is persistence of HPV infection or reinfection by a new sexual partner. When a lesion is discovered by this close follow-up monitoring, then typically the same treatment protocol as was discussed in each scenario before will be administered.

There are clinical situations in which the extent of a high-grade lesion is such that both LEEP and cold-knife cone procedures are unable to remove it all. This presents a very difficult management choice for women who still wish to have children. This clinical scenario is difficult enough that making recommendations in this book would not be appropriate. It requires a complex and highly individualized management scheme that is best left up to a gynecologic oncologist—a gynecologist who specializes in cancer treatment.

If the patient has no desire to have additional children, then often a complete hysterectomy will be advised.

We'll look at this more extensively in the next chapter.

7

If You Have Cancer

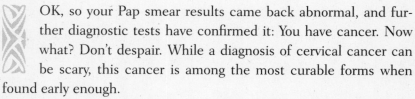 OK, so your Pap smear results came back abnormal, and further diagnostic tests have confirmed it: You have cancer. Now what? Don't despair. While a diagnosis of cervical cancer can be scary, this cancer is among the most curable forms when found early enough.

This chapter is a brief look at treatment options for those with cancer. Its purpose is to give you an introduction to some of the basic issues that arise in the treatment of cervical, vaginal, and vulvar cancer and to point you in the direction of other helpful resources.

SYMPTOMS OF INVASIVE CERVICAL CANCER

Early cervical cancer does not cause any symptoms. This may sound peculiar, considering the drama that's taking place on a cellular level within your body, but remember that this is a microdrama. You experience only macroevents. You do not notice, for example, your skin cells being born, rising to the surface, dying, and being sloughed off, although this takes place continuously throughout your life. Nor can you observe that process with the naked eye. Similarly, the abnormal growth of cells won't be noticeable even after it penetrates the basement membrane. Your cells may be proliferating like maniacs, but you don't know it. Unfortunately, often when there are symptoms, it indicates more advanced disease.

When cervical cancer becomes invasive, you may experience pain during intercourse, bleeding beyond your period, or unusual discharge. If you are experiencing any of these symptoms, don't delay. Seek help now! There may be other, more benign explanations for these symptoms, such as hormonal changes or yeast infection, for example, but don't assume that these benign causes provide the explanation for your symptoms. Be sure to check with your health-care provider and get a definitive diagnosis, no matter what your age. If you're a young woman, don't assume that cervical cancer affects only older people. Remember that the age of girls affected by HPV is growing ever younger and that this virus can lead to invasive cervical cancer. If you're a middle-aged woman, don't dismiss these symptoms by telling yourself "I'm probably just going through menopause." And if you're an older woman, don't ignore them because you're monogamous and think that you can't be affected by this disease. Fifteen years ago, when I was in medical school, the profile of the typical cervical cancer patient was a woman in her late forties and older. Unfortunately, now, as Kate's story illustrates, deaths in the early thirties are a hard, cold reality.

THE ROLE OF THE PATHOLOGIST AFTER DIAGNOSIS

Until now, we have been discussing the role of the pathologist in looking at Pap smears and biopsies to determine if there is a precancerous or cancerous process going on. After an invasive cancer is discovered, my role certainly does not cease. It is the pathologist's job to examine invasive cancer specimens and provide key information about the disease. This information then guides the type of therapy selected. The most important pieces of information a pathologist must provide about an invasive cancer are the *type, grade,* and *stage* of the cancer.

DETERMINING THE TYPE OF CANCER PRESENT

Certainly, to begin with, the first step is to identify the type of cancer we're dealing with. The two major types involved in cervical cancer are squamous carcinoma and adenocarcinoma. These two types behave somewhat differently. In addition to these two major types, there are a small number of very rare types of cervical cancer, some of which have no relationship to HPV at all. These must be assessed and identified, since they also have different behaviors.

DETERMINING THE GRADE OF CANCER

The "grade" of a cancer is a term we use to communicate how aggressive the cancer appears to be, using certain microscopic features. These microscopic features include how much the cancer looks like the original cells from which it was derived. That's called the *differentiation* of the cancer. The grade is expressed according to how well differentiated the cancer is. The more an invasive cancer looks like the original cells, the less aggressive it's likely to be. This is called a *well-*

differentiated cancer. On the other end of the spectrum, an invasive cancer that bears little if any resemblance to the type of cells from which is was derived is called a *poorly differentiated cancer* and tends to behave much more aggressively.

Another important feature in the grading of a cancer is assessing how fast it is multiplying. Obviously, a cancer that is dividing more rapidly will probably behave more aggressively than one dividing more slowly.

DETERMINING THE STAGE OF CANCER

"Stage" is a term used to communicate how large a cancer is and how far it has extended. Cancers that are caught very early—in other words, just after they have begun to cross the basement membrane—are called *low-stage cancers.* Cancers that have spread very far into surrounding organs and lymph nodes are *high-stage cancers.* The current accepted staging system for all cancers of the female genitalia is called the *FIGO (Federation of International Gynecologic Oncology) Staging System.* This system is quite complicated, containing far more categories than merely the two we have discussed—"low-stage" and "high-stage." It is a numerical system requiring a great deal of information, in part provided by the pathologist, about the extent of the cancer.

Once a pathologist has provided all of this accurate information, the next steps can be taken by a team of surgeons who specialize in female cancers—*gynecologic oncologists*—and physicians who specialize in radiation treatment, called *radiation oncologists.* The most effective treatment plans for the therapy of any gynecologic cancer results from numerous conferences between pathologists, gynecologic oncologists, and radiation oncologists so that an individualized treatment plan can be designed.

Now let's look at the components of most treatment plans and what you might expect from each.

First of All, Get Treatment!

It may surprise you to learn that many women diagnosed with cervical cancer never pursue treatment. A study conducted by the National Cancer Institute found that 10 percent of patients diagnosed with early-stage disease never pursued treatment after receiving their diagnosis. Among patients with advanced disease, the numbers were even higher. The largest number of untreated patients were over sixty-five years old.

These statistics are baffling to me. Cervical cancer has one of the highest cure rates when it's treated early—about 90 percent. And even for more advanced cases, there is a 50-percent cure rate. I don't understand why affected women would walk away from life-saving treatment.

Dr. Edward Trimble of the National Cancer Institute, who conducted the study, suggested that some women are afraid of the treatment protocol—especially radiation—and that some patients may not be sufficiently informed about what it entails. The purpose of this chapter is to provide you with some education regarding treatments so you are motivated, well informed, and committed to your treatment plan.

Your treatment plan will probably consist of surgery, radiation, or some combination of both. These have been mainstays of cervical cancer treatment for over half a century. More recently, chemotherapy has been added to the mix, but usually for higher stage disease. Over these years, and right to this day, active debate and research continue regarding just which and how much of each modality to use for each type, stage, and grade of cancer.

Very recently, Americans have begun to search for alternatives to these three pillars of cancer therapy. Some of these alternatives can be effective and useful, especially in helping patients to reduce the side effects of conventional treatments and build their general state of health so that the body's own healing mechanisms can aid in the process of fighting cancer. Certainly, the emotional and spiritual elements are usually given more careful attention by less-conventional practitioners. Sadly, however, there is a great deal of misinformation and many quacks in the world of alternative medicine. Many are not knowledgeable and are highly irresponsible. It is often hard for the consumer to distinguish between authentic and inauthentic remedies and healers. Dr. Warshowsky will discuss safe and responsible complementary approaches in greater detail in Chapter 10 and will help you incorporate them into a healing program. Additional reliable resources will be available at the end of this book.

As with other fields of medicine, treatment of cervical cancer is in a state of constant growth and evolution. But take comfort in the fact that these therapies have progressed to the point that more than 80 percent of early-stage invasive cervical cancers are curable.

RADIOTHERAPY

Radiation has, since its discovery, been one of our strongest weapons in the fight against cancer. The principle is simple: radiation, as we all know from the results of Hiroshima and Chernobyl, is a killer. Radiation kills by damaging cellular DNA. In massive doses, it will kill the whole body. But if the radiation is controlled in its strength and directed to the site of a cancer like a laser beam, it can effectively destroy a cancer and spare the rest of the body.

The radiation can be delivered to the affected cancerous site with an external beam, which is not invasive and is similar to getting a chest X ray. Another method places the source of radiation very close to the cancer, usually by some form of implanted internal device.

Cervical cancer is one of the few cancers that in earlier stages can be completely treated by radiotherapy. In more advanced stages, radiotherapy can also be used to control the spread of the disease. The most common method of irradiating a cervical cancer is to use an internal device placed in the vagina next to the cervix. This device delivers high-energy radiation directly to this relatively limited area. Although effective, this treatment method is, like all treatment methods, not free of side effects. Side effects of local radiation can include urinary, rectal, and intestinal problems, as well as difficulty maintaining cervical and vaginal lubrication. While these side effects often disappear once the treatment is over, some may persist long after the cancer has been cured. A number of additional medications, exercises, and other remedies are available to alleviate these symptoms. These should be discussed with your health-care provider. Often, the nursing staff is also familiar with ways to minimize or deal with side effects. Additional suggestions can be found in the Resources section of this book.

SURGERY

The principle behind surgery is even simpler than the principle behind radiation. If there's a cancer, cut it out! This is the principle behind the previously discussed cone biopsies—they are used for diagnosis and to play it safe. The lesion is removed in case it is cancerous. In more advanced stage cervical cancers, more extensive surgery is the primary option. As stated earlier, there is still considerable debate about the role of surgery in earlier stage cancers. Again, these decisions must be individualized for each patient.

The essential surgical procedure used for invasive cervical cancer is called a *hysterectomy,* which is the surgical removal of the uterus and its attached cervix. Not all hysterectomies are the same. Indeed, various types of hysterectomy are performed for various stages of cervical cancer. The difference in these procedures generally involves how much of the tissues around the uterus are removed together with the uterus. Obviously, more advanced cancers will require removal of more tissues than earlier stage cancers.

The most extensive hysterectomies involve the removal of the uterus and cervix, all of the surrounding ligaments, the upper portion of the vagina, and all of the lymph nodes that serve the area. In extremely advanced cases of cervical cancer—cases in which the cancer has spread to involve the neighboring structures of the bladder and rectum—an even more aggressive excision of all these structures may be chosen.

Sometimes removal of the ovaries is necessary as well, though even in the most advanced cases, for reasons that are unclear, cervical cancer rarely spreads to the ovaries. As we discussed in Chapter 2, the ovaries are the primary source of important female hormones such as estrogen and progesterone. Removal of the ovaries plunges women into *surgical menopause*. The symptoms can be even more severe than those associated with natural menopause because the hormones produced by the ovaries have been removed suddenly, instead of dwindling gradually as the woman ages. For this reason, particularly in younger women who have not yet gone through menopause, attempts are made to spare the ovaries.

Aside from the challenge of dealing with cancer, the adjustment to life without a uterus can be formidable. If you are a young woman, you may be dealing with the additional issue of being infertile. It is essential that you work closely with your health-care provider to help you through this difficult period. You may need hormone replacement therapy of some kind to help rebalance your hormones after the procedure, even if your ovaries have been left intact. Alternative health approaches, including herbs, acupuncture, and mind-body techniques may be helpful. Some counseling or couple's therapy might be of help if the procedure has adversely affected your intimate life.

CHEMOTHERAPY

In chemotherapy, powerful drugs are used to kill the cancer cells. They are designed to interfere with the process of cell division so the cancer can't continue replicating itself. These chemicals can kill healthy as well as diseased tissue. The dosage needs careful adjustment so that it is strong enough to be effective against the cancer, but not so strong that it kills the entire body. As I said above, chemotherapy is a relative latecomer in the treatment of cervical cancer and is typically reserved for advanced stage disease. There is considerable debate regarding how effective it may be in various situations. Your doctor will decide if it is appropriate for you.

Most people are familiar with the side effects of chemotherapy, which include fatigue, nausea, hair loss, depression and mood swings, body aches, and general malaise. Although these side effects disappear once the chemotherapy has run its course, they are extremely unpleasant and augment the already formidable challenges of dealing with having cancer to begin with, and with the effects of surgery. Fortunately, in the last five years, a number of new drugs have been developed to alleviate some of these side effects.

Handling the negative effects of chemotherapy requires a multimodal approach that combines psychological support and symptomatic relief. Chapter 10 will introduce you to alternative modalities such as herbs and acupuncture that might alleviate some of the symptoms.

Vulvar and Vaginal Cancers

Most cancers of the vulva and vagina are also caused by high-risk strains of HPV. Vaginal cancers often manifest with similar symptoms to cervical cancer—bleeding and pain during intercourse. While the Pap smear may pick up a few vaginal cells, it won't test for vulvar cancer. However, Pap smears are not necessary for the detection of vulvar cancers because these external lesions are usually discovered by the patient or through visual examination by her gynecologist. They can look like irritated or ulcerated sores, readily visible to the eye. A biopsy is performed to confirm a diagnosis of cancer.

Treatment for vulvar cancer has evolved considerably in recent years. Surgery used to be drastic, and involved removal of the vulva, lymph nodes, clitoris, and labia. Today, surgeons prefer to remove as little as possible, trying to preserve the clitoris and labia. They use skin grafts from other parts of the body to rebuild the area if possible.

The type of *vulvectomy* (removal of the vulva) performed depends on whether the cancer has spread, to what regions it has spread, and how far it has spread. Surgery may be followed by radiation or chemotherapy.

Treatment of vaginal cancer also depends on the extent of the disease and how far it has spread. Options range from *vaginectomy* (removal of the vagina) to laser therapy, *intravaginal chemotherapy* (chemotherapy applied directly to the vagina), or radiation. Sometimes more than one of these is used.

The sexual repercussions of both vulvar and vaginal cancer are far more difficult to deal with than those connected with cervical cancer. But they can be overcome, and you can continue to enjoy intimacy with your partner. You and your partner will need to learn new ways to give each other pleasure. You'll need to be open with communication, and you'll need to be creative. Enlisting the assistance of a professional, such as a sex therapist or nurse with a specialty in dealing with women's oncological issues, will be very helpful.

DEALING WITH CANCER

There is probably no more dreaded disease in this country than cancer, and with good reason. Cancer has claimed the lives of millions of people, exacting from them great suffering first. But cancer is no longer a death sentence. Researchers have begun to understand how this terrible disease works and have begun to find powerful new medications to reverse it or at least to slow its progress. Nor do people have to suffer in isolation. Libraries, bookstores, and the Internet abound with excellent resources to help cancer patients and their families deal with the practical, as well as the emotional, implications of the disease. Most major cities have support groups run by hospitals, churches, or community centers to help cancer patients and their families, and most mental health centers and hospitals have mental health professionals who are trained to help patients work through the myriad of difficult issues that arise.

This chapter was designed to provide you with some basic information about what happens if you develop a cancer of the genital region. In addition to Dr. Warshowsky's advice in Chapter 10, I have included an extensive list of resources and suggestions for further reading at the back of this book. I strongly urge you to avail yourself of the rich array of support and resources during this difficult time. Most of all, I again urge you to seek treatment for this often-curable cancer.

8

Genital Warts

 So far we have concentrated primarily on cervical cancer as the most dangerous outcome of HPV, though throughout this book, we have alluded to genital warts. This chapter will take a look at genital warts in greater detail, focusing on how you can identify and treat them—and, hopefully, prevent their recurrence.

MY INTRODUCTION TO GENITAL WARTS AND HPV

When I was medical student, I was asked to examine a fifteen-year-old girl. I had been conducting examinations for several months by then and was beginning to regard myself as something of an old pro.

I entered the examination room and saw a young girl clearly in distress. Her boyfriend was standing next to her, holding her hand.

"What seems to be the problem?" I asked the patient.

She fumbled for words. "Something is wrong with my—I mean, I've got this problem, you know, and it's getting in the way of, well, you know." She pointed. It emerged that she was seeking treatment because she and her boyfriend could no longer have intercourse due to some problem in her genital area.

When I examined the area, all my newly discovered professional composure fled. Her vulva was covered by enormous cauliflowerlike growths. The warts were so extensive I couldn't even get a speculum into her vagina. I managed to mumble something about needing "another opinion" and hurried out of the room. I located one of the senior ob/gyn residents. After she examined the girl, I received my first lecture on genital warts and HPV.

What Are Genital Warts?

Genital warts can appear on the vagina, vulva, or cervix in women, and the shaft or head of the penis in men. They can appear around the anus and urethra in both men and women.

Most of us have an idea of what a typical wart looks like, based on our experiences with warts on the finger or foot. A wart on your finger is usually a round, brownish, somewhat raised spot. However, warts can also be white and spiky in appearance. The warts in the genital area can look similar. But unfortunately, they don't always conform to this image. In fact, they can often be completely flat and invisible to the naked eye. Sometimes, they are flat and pigmented, looking like a lightly colored mole.

Flat lesions aren't the only warts that are hard to detect. Even classic raised lesions are challenging because they are often very small and blend in almost seamlessly with the skin in the genitalia, which naturally has a finely nodular texture. So if you're thinking that a quick way to prevent HPV infection is to inspect your partner's genitalia for warts, think again. These lesions can be invisible even to trained physicians. Moreover, these warts may be internal. They may be present in the urethra of both men and women, and in the vagina and cervix. These are areas you can't really inspect visually.

Genital warts are usually painless. However, sometimes they may become sore. They may itch or burn—especially if they're ignored for a long time, or if they've been rubbed. Sexual activity can be an irritant because of the rubbing and massaging involved. As warts multiply and spread throughout the region, they can sometimes cause incontinence.

Genital warts, even when small, can be cosmetically unappealing to the affected individual as well as to the partner. And obviously, severe cases of rampant genital warts such as I encountered in my patient while I was in medical school are not only a cosmetic problem but also a medical problem. They obstruct the urethra so that the patient can't urinate. This is a problem especially for men, who often come for treatment because they are unable to void.

Extensive warts can also obstruct the vagina. This impedes sexual intercourse, as it did in the case of my young, distressed patient. And if this doesn't sound awful enough, the most serious outcome is the development of cancer. These cancers can develop anywhere in the genital and the anal areas of both females and males. Remember that genital warts can be caused by low-risk as well as high-risk viral strains. Low-risk viruses are usually responsible for the more florid and oversized genital warts. High-risk viruses can also cause warty lesions, but more often result in the so-called flat wart. Just as in the cervix, infection with the high-risk HPV types can result in invasive squamous cell cancer, depending on the "deal" the virus works out with the cells, and the strength or weakness of the immune system.

Flat warts, in particular, are more commonly associated with various forms of cancer. They are often called vulvar intraepithelial neoplasia (VIN1) and play a similar role in vulvar cancer to LGSIL in cervical cancer. They are also responsible for higher-grade cancers of the vulvar, vaginal, anal, and penile areas. As they advance through the levels of premalignancy, they can become very red or even blacken.

DIAGNOSING GENITAL WARTS

The diagnosis of genital warts needs to be done by a trained health-care provider—typically, a gynecologist, dermatologist, or trained family practitioner. Genital warts are usually diagnosed with a visual examination. To find hard-to-detect warts, your health-care provider will soak suspicious areas with a dilute acetic acid solution to look for whitening that's typical of wart tissue. To locate very small warts, it may be necessary to use a strong magnifying instrument during examination of the genital area. Some doctors will have to examine a small sample of tissue under a microscope to dispel any further doubts.

Your doctor may order a biopsy, depending on the appearance, location, and responsiveness of your lesions. If there is any doubt about whether a suspicious area is due to a recent injury or some other inflammatory skin condition, for example, a biopsy will be helpful in determining the nature of the lesion. If you're being treated for genital warts but they are not responding, your doctor may order a biopsy to investigate why this is the case.

TREATING GENITAL WARTS

There are many different types of treatment for genital warts, depending on the size and location of the wart, and how extensive the infection is. There is no single treatment protocol, and different health-care practitioners seem to have their own preferences regarding which modality or medicine they start with and how they proceed. Here are the various possibilities:

CHEMICAL TREATMENTS

There is an array of chemical agents called *cytotoxins,* designed to "poison" the cells in the wart. They are applied directly to the wart by your health-care provider in the office over several sessions on a scheduled basis. They include the following:

Podophyllin

Podophyllin is a medication derived from mayapples. Because it can cause neurological side effects, physicians generally try to avoid applying it to large areas so that the body won't absorb excessive quantities. If you are treated with podophyllin, be sure to wash the treated area four to six hours after treatment—and sooner if you experience discomfort. Although it's not usually painful during application, it can cause significant discomfort for several days afterward. It should not be used in the vagina, urethra, or cervix and should be avoided during pregnancy.

Podophyllotoxin

Podophyllotoxin is a less toxic cousin of podophyllin. It's applied by the patient rather than by the doctor, and it does not have the potentially dangerous side effects associated with podophyllin. Some people experience mild skin irritation. About 75 percent of those treated with podophyllotoxin will respond, but about one-third of these cases will experience a recurrence.

5-Fluorouracil (5-FU) Cream

This cream is used particularly to treat vaginal, anal, urethral, and vulvar warts. It works by addressing the lesion at the DNA level. It's been associated with some serious side effects, including severe inflammation and pain as well as malformation of the fetus in pregnant women, so most practitioners try to avoid it.

Trichloroacetic Acid (TCA) and Bichloroacetic Acid (BCA)
These are probably the most useful and popular chemical agents. They are also inexpensive, which is an added benefit. They are used to treat vulvar, anal, penile, vaginal, and urethral warts, and are applied by the physician. The downside is that momentary burning occurs when the solution is applied to the lesion. Unfortunately, any spillover can burn healthy surrounding areas seriously and the pain can last for several hours. So it's impractical to treat a large area in a single visit, and you might be asked to return once or twice a week until the warts go away or another treatment method is sought. Lidocaine ointment and ice packs can provide relief of the pain. TCA and BCA are absorbed only in the skin, so they are safe for use during pregnancy. Don't worry if you notice a shallow ulcer—a little hole—left behind after the wart has been sloughed off. That's normal and will clear up within a couple of weeks.

SURGERY

Surgical treatment of genital warts can take many different forms. Most can be performed in the doctor's office with local anesthesia. However, because the problem lies in the presence of the virus within the system, warts are likely to return unless the deeper immune issues are addressed.

Cryotherapy
In this procedure, liquid nitrogen is placed directly on the wart and a small area of surrounding skin, which freezes the area. Small ice crystals are formed, killing all of the epithelial cells in the area, thus causing the wart to slough off. Cryotherapy can be used for warts on most areas, including the cervix, but should not be used within the vagina. Some women complain about extreme discomfort during treatment

due to the cold. Don't be too shy to ask for a topical anesthetic cream if you feel uncomfortable. Be reassured that the pain is usually short-lived—a few days at most—and does not last through the whole healing period. Cryotherapy is administered at weekly intervals. Clearance rates of the warts is quite high (90 percent) and some additional chemical therapy enhances the success of this method.

Electrosurgery

This is a procedure using an instrument similar to that described for LEEP in which an electrified instrument is used to remove the wart and control local bleeding at the same time. This procedure is still employed by some practitioners because the equipment is relatively inexpensive, although laser vaporization is regarded as superior. Small areas can be treated using local anesthetic, but treatment of a larger area requires general anesthetic. Because the equipment is less expensive than laser, electrosurgery is certainly the most cost-efficient approach to treating warts when they resist topical chemical agents. Unlike with laser, electrosurgery can cause burns, although permanent scarring is unusual. Although all the warts can be removed during a single treatment, about 20 to 30 percent of the warts will recur and necessitate further treatment.

Scissor Excision

This procedure involves using a sharp instrument to manually cut out the wart. It might be useful when there are a very small number of isolated warts or when the practitioner would like to send the wart to a laboratory for a biopsy. It is not effective for large numbers of warts, and those that are removed tend to recur.

Laser Vaporization

In this procedure, an intense light beam is used to destroy the warts. It was the mainstay of treatment of severe external genital warts as well as intraepithelial lesions. However, because of practical issues such as the high cost of equipment and the extensive training required to learn the technique, it tends to be reserved for only the most complicated cases. It is an extremely precise and effective treatment, particularly useful in treating large external lesions or lesions that appear in areas that are hard to reach, such as the vagina, anus, and the vaginal crevices located in the vestibule. The cure rates are similar to those of electrosurgery. Some 20 to 30 percent of the warts will recur, necessitating further treatment.

IMMUNOTHERAPY

Immunotherapy is the boosting of the immune system to help it heal the body itself. It is used either as a stand-alone primary treatment or together with chemical or surgical approaches. The treatments discussed below are all immunotherapeutic.

Interferon

Interferon is an antiviral drug that is injected directly into the warts. It is a chemical released by the immune system to defend against invading viruses. However, it is expensive and difficult to administer. Moreover, it causes unpleasant side effects, such as fever, muscle aches, and flulike symptoms.

Imiquimod

Imiquimod promotes a natural but somewhat enhanced immune response to HPV. Since warts recur because the body's immune system is unable to suppress the virus, Imiquimod is especially useful after the lesions have been removed in preventing recurrence by stimulating immune response. It is applied by the patient directly to the where the wart was before removal three times a week for eight to ten weeks. Imiquimod has an excellent success rate in promoting clearance of warts and preventing them from returning.

Your Partner Should Be Treated, Too

If you have an STD, your partner almost certainly has it too. It doesn't matter who gave it to whom first—diseases don't come with a return address. And if you've been faithful, don't rush to suspect that he has had an affair. I don't want you hitting him over the head with this book! As we know, HPV can lie latent for many years. He might have gotten it from his high school girlfriend and has been carrying it around for a decade or two. Remember that you can have HPV without any obvious symptoms. And even if he develops noticeable warts, the latent virus might suddenly be reactivated due to aging, stress, poor diet, or any of the other factors described elsewhere in this book.

One thing is clear: You both need to be treated. Even if your partner doesn't have any obvious-looking warts, he must see a health-care professional. As we discussed earlier in this chapter, flat warts are exceedingly difficult to spot, even by seasoned experts. They're even easier for a lay person to miss. Moreover, they're even easier to miss in men because they can grow less aggressively and blatantly on the penis, which is drier than the vulvar area in women. If you have HPV, your partner should see his health-care provider who may conduct a more extensive test than merely a visual exam. So don't make assumptions. Send him for treatment.

The treatments described in this chapter are really nothing more than stopgap measures. They jump-start a process of healing that is longer and more complex. Remember that none of these approaches guarantees that the warts will not return. Once you have the virus, it inhabits the entire region, even areas that don't produce any symptoms. The lifestyle tips offered in Chapters 10 and 11 are your best bet for building your immune system and enhancing your body's ability to fight the virus.

9

Not for Women Only—HPV, Men, and Children

After reading earlier chapters of this book, perhaps you've been left with a sense of resentment and injustice. How unfair that this virus should cause such extensive damage in women, while leaving men relatively unaffected! There is some measure of truth to your perception. HPV seems to be an equal-opportunity infector, but not an equal-opportunity afflicter. Still, men can also be seriously affected.

Although cervical cancer obviously affects only women (men don't have cervices), HPV affects everybody. I'm not referring here to plantar warts. We all know that men, women, and children can get warts on their fingers and feet. But it may surprise you to know that sexually transmitted forms of HPV can affect people of all ages and genders, including those who are not sexually active. Even stranger, it can affect regions of the body other than the genitals. Let's look at how that works.

OF LOCKS AND KEYS

Remember our discussion in Chapter 1 of the different strains of HPV and how specific they are? I said that women do not need to worry that a wart on their partner's foot can infect their genital region with HPV. I explained that the various strains of HPV are highly specific and that their ligands need specific receptors, not all of which are equally present in all parts of the body. So the strain that likes to latch on to feet is not likely to latch on to the cervical area.

However, there are certain strains that like the other epithelial linings of the body. Remember that the female reproductive tract, the anus, throat, nasal passages, bronchi, larynx, and the tubes within the lungs are all covered by epithelial lining. Obviously, these body parts are not exclusive to women. Additionally, a woman's infection can also spread to her partner's penis. And a pregnant woman can sometimes communicate the infection to the respiratory tract of her baby.

HOW HPV AFFECTS MEN

During sex—even with a condom—the exposed area of the man's genitals (the base of his penis and his scrotum) can contract HPV from contact with his partner. Condoms do not cover these areas. Depending on the strain of the virus, he can develop either condyloma lesions—large, cauliflowerlike growths—in those areas, or he can develop flat, less-detectable warts. Because of the highly contagious nature of the virus, these can spread to other areas, including the penis and the anus. Often, men are infected with the virus without ever showing symptoms. Far more men than women carry the virus without knowing they have it. In scientific terms, they are called *asympto-*

matic carriers. It is these men who are probably responsible for the spread of the disease because their lesions are not detectable.

As in women, HPV can take a more insidious turn than merely confining itself to unpleasant warts. Men are also susceptible to cancers. Penile cancer, though rare, can be an outcome of HPV infection. Although there are only 1,200 new cases reported annually in the United States, it is a much more common ailment in other parts of the world, such as the African countries. The mechanism of development of penile cancer follows the same general principles as those discussed regarding cervical and vulvar carcinoma. Infection by high-risk viral types, followed by a series of events in the DNA and the failure of the immune system to kick in, can lead to the same invasive squamous carcinoma as in women. You may ask yourself, then: If the same mechanism is involved, why is this so much rarer in men? Scientists have not yet arrived at a conclusive answer to this question, but part of the answer may be that the penis has no transformation zone.

Men also can suffer from anal cancer. Precancerous anal dysplasia is similar to precancerous cervical dysplasia. HPV has been found in anal lesions, just as it has in cervical lesions, and the same strains of virus are responsible for high-grade lesions in both areas. Be aware that women are as susceptible to anal lesions as men are. Remember our discussion of the squamocolumnar junction in Chapter 2? Like the cervix, the anal canal has a squamocolumnar junction, where the squamous epithelial cells meet the columnar cells. This is the site where the most severe disease strikes.

HPV is also frequently transmitted through homosexual intercourse. Prior to the emergence of the HIV epidemic, the incidence of anal cancer in gay men was estimated to be about 35 cases per 100,000. (Interestingly, this is identical to the incidence of cervical cancer prior to the routine use of Pap smears.) It is estimated that today, this number has doubled. Indeed, in some areas of the country with a large male homosexual population, health-care practitioners have begun to employ anal Pap smears to screen for the possible development of anal cancer.

Symptoms of penile and anal cancer are similar to those described for vulvar cancer. Both types of cancers can manifest in one of two ways: One is the appearance of a chronic ulcer that continues to grow larger without healing and often bleeds. The second is a large wartlike lesion that continues to grow over time. Because of this, any lesions you see or feel or any episodes of chronic rectal bleeding should be immediately investigated by your physician—particularly if you are also affected by genital warts.

Treatment of external warts or precancerous conditions in the male genital tract is similar to treatment of the condition in the female genital tract. If you think that your partner may be affected, encourage him to consult with a primary care physician or urologist.

HPV AND PREGNANCY

As you will see in the next section, children can sometimes contract HPV from their mothers during childbirth. Does this mean that if you have ever been diagnosed with HPV, or have suffered from any of the conditions associated with HPV, such as genital warts or cervical dysplasia, you should never have children? Current thinking is that it is safe to become pregnant. It is unlikely that you will communicate the virus to your baby during pregnancy. But inform your obstetrician because, as we will see in the next section, childbirth appears to be the crucial time of transmission. Studies show that children of HPV-infected mothers who have been delivered by cesarean section are less likely to contract the disease. Although a C-section for an HPV-infected mother is not standard of care as of this writing, I believe that it is wise to err on the side of caution here and at least consider this option. As you will see below, the consequences of transmitting the virus to an infant can be serious and even deadly.

HPV AND CHILDREN

During the last few years, there has been a disturbing increase in the number of young children between the ages of two and five years old turning up in emergency rooms with *stridor.* "Stridor" means noisy breathing, and it can be caused by many different types of respiratory ailments. A patient with stridor has obstructed air passages, causing a wheezing, crowing, or howling noise when the patient attempts to breathe. In very severe cases, the airways become so obstructed that no breath can enter or exit and the patient suffocates.

It turned out that many of these children are suffering from *recurrent respiratory papillomatosis,* which is caused by HPV infection of the respiratory tract—usually with types 6 and 11. These are low-risk viruses when it comes to cancer, but are responsible for warts. And in fact, that is what these children have. In this disease, large warty lesions, called *papillomas,* grow within the respiratory tract of children. They can be present in the mouth, throat, and vocal cords and can extend even as far as the lungs.

How, you may ask, could children possibly get this horrendous manifestation of HPV infection? As far back as 1956, an astute pediatrician named Hajek observed that often children who developed these lesions were born to mothers with genital warts. Another very important finding was made by Dr. K. Shah, probably the foremost HPV researcher in the world, when he studied over 100 children with this disease and found that only one was born by cesarean section. Since then, it has become clear through multiple studies that a major mechanism of infection by HPV is *vertical transmission,* or transmission of the virus from pregnant mother to infant. It is believed that when a baby passes through the cervix, vagina, and vulva of an HPV-infected woman during childbirth, the virus invades the baby's respiratory tract. Remember that HPV is communicated through skin-to-skin contact. During childbirth, the infant passes through the birth canal and is therefore in intimate contact with the infected areas of the mother's cervix, vagina, and vulva. HPV-laden cells enter the baby's mouth and nostrils. This can be the case, even if the mother is not showing any symptoms of HPV infection. Usually, the virus remains latent for several years and then, for reasons still poorly understood, begins acting up when the child is about three years old. It is possible that the lesions have been growing slowly during that entire time and only reach a critical mass after a few years.

It is also unclear why some children born to HPV-infected mothers contract this condition while most do not. Some evidence suggests that the dynamics at play here in determining who will become symptomatic and who won't are similar to those that affect adults. These include such factors as smoking, nutrition, and the strength of the mother's and child's immune system.

Perhaps the worst aspect of this condition is that it is recurrent. I have seen kids whose childhoods are punctuated by repeated emergency room trips due to obstructed airways and repeated surgical procedures to remove the lesions. These frequent recurrences of the disease and the necessary surgery can cause chronic inflammation and permanent damage to the vocal cords. Children with respiratory papillomatosis have an average of four surgical treatments each year to remove lesions, but some children require surgery every two to three weeks!

The toll this takes on the child is not only physical. The psychological repercussions of constant illness and rounds of surgery are traumatic and impede a child's possibility of enjoying a normal childhood. And the price paid by the family—emotional as well as financial—is staggering.

Children can die of respiratory papillomatosis when the airway is so obstructed that the emergency room staff are unable to *intubate,* or insert a tube into the airway to facilitate airflow, or when the lesions spread to lung tissue. Between 1 and 3 percent of children with this condition die.

Respiratory papillomatosis is an equal-opportunity afflicter. No ethnic or racial group is immune. One study of 399 children with this condition found that 63 percent were Caucasian, 28 percent were African-American, and 11 percent were Hispanic. The children were evenly divided by gender. It is estimated that in 1999, there might have been as many as 1,500 new cases, with as many as 3,000 children affected. This number has increased during the three years since that conservative estimate was offered.

With the alarming rise in cases of HPV, we can probably expect to see the number of affected children increase sharply. Certainly, this is what my colleagues who work in emergency rooms and specialize in the surgical removal of these lesions tell me.

Immunotheraphy, particularly with interferon, has been tried, with some success, but there is still a high recurrence rate with this drug. A new nonprescription drug made from indole-3-carbinol (I3C), which is a naturally occurring chemical in cruciferous vegetables such as broccoli, seems to have a remarkable effect on a significant number of patients. A recent clinical trial showed remission in a third of patients, a slow growth rate in another third, and no response in the last third. Additional studies of this promising drug are underway.

Sadly, public health officials have not paid sufficient attention to this problem—possibly because an insufficient number of people have died from it, and it's not considered worthy of attention and a massive public campaign. But we don't want more children to die of a preventable illness! This is an opportunity for teachers and school nurses to talk to children, for doctors and health professionals to talk to patients, and for friends to talk to friends so that, at the very least, information about juvenile respiratory papillomatosis can be spread by word of mouth—indeed, much like the spreading of a virus. Let's make education and informed health care a national epidemic.

One last word on HPV and children. In the past, the presence of lesions in the genital or anal areas of a young child was considered a sure-fire sign of sexual abuse. How else would the virus reach such an intimate area of the body? Today, the thinking has shifted somewhat. Although sexual molestation is still the most likely explanation and should be thoroughly investigated, it is possible that the virus was communicated to the child during childbirth and has appeared in the genital tract rather than the respiratory tract several years later. If proper precautions are taken during childbirth, however, respiratory papillomatosis is entirely preventable in children.

10

HPV and Cervical Disease—A Holistic Approach
by Allan Warshowsky, M.D.

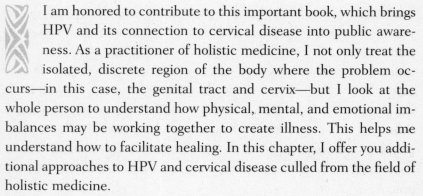 I am honored to contribute to this important book, which brings HPV and its connection to cervical disease into public awareness. As a practitioner of holistic medicine, I not only treat the isolated, discrete region of the body where the problem occurs—in this case, the genital tract and cervix—but I look at the whole person to understand how physical, mental, and emotional imbalances may be working together to create illness. This helps me understand how to facilitate healing. In this chapter, I offer you additional approaches to HPV and cervical disease culled from the field of holistic medicine.

Before we look at specifics of HPV and cervical disease, I'd like to take a somewhat more in-depth look at holistic medicine. Perhaps the best way to begin is to tell you how I became interested in holistic medicine.

I am a board-certified gynecologist. In medical school back in the 1970s, I became disheartened by some of the limitations of the medical approaches I was studying—specifically, medicine's inability to help those with chronic illnesses. That feeling stayed with me even after I opened my own practice. I kept thinking that there must be something that could help women with supposedly incurable and chronic conditions.

I began to spend more time listening to my patients and learning about their lives, not merely about their medical conditions. In working with the condition known as premenstrual syndrome, I was disturbed to discover that some patients' complaints had never been taken seriously before, and some patients felt they had never really been *heard* by a doctor. An article I read about vitamins inspired me to research them, and I began suggesting that my patients take basic vitamin supplements. To my surprise, I had great success in helping them to alleviate some of their symptoms. Soon, compassionate listening and vitamin supplementation became as important to my treatment protocols as pharmaceuticals and surgery.

I was going through my own personal life changes at this time and was attending personal growth workshops. I began to realize that it was artificial to separate my personal perspectives from my professional perspectives. The techniques of active listening and the attitude of regarding mind, body, and spirit as an interconnected web essential to healing became important in my practice as well as in my personal life. I expanded my attendance at workshops to include those focusing on the immune system, on non-Western medical approaches to illness and health, on herbs, and on other aspects of health and healing. I incorporated my newfound knowledge into my practice of obstetrics and gynecology.

It was gratifying to witness the many positive changes in the lives and health of my patients—and equally gratifying to see how many patients were interested in taking a holistic approach to their health. When I was affiliated with Long Island Jewish Hospital, about 60 to 75 percent of my practice consisted of patients who chose me as their physician specifically because they wanted a holistic approach. They liked my focus on building health, not only on curing sickness. They liked the range of conventional and complementary modalities that I offered. Now, as the director of the Women's Program at the Continuum Center for Health and Healing of the Beth Israel Hospital in Manhattan, all of my patients come to me because they are looking for this approach. And they are not alone. Recent studies show that an increasing number of Americans are exploring alternative approaches to their health problems. It is estimated that in 1998, 69 percent of Americans used some form of alternative medicine—up from 34 percent in 1990. Alternative practitioners logged 629 million visits in 1997.

Among physicians, the word is also spreading. I became involved with the American Holistic Medical Association—an organization consisting of more than 900 medical doctors and osteopaths—which helped to shape my understanding of what holistic medicine is and what it is not.

Holistic medicine doesn't just involve finding an herbal substitute for a conventional drug and using it to treat a disease, or using vitamins and nutritional supplements to build health and strengthen immunity. The holistic approach embraces all facets of the human being—mind, body, and spirit. An imbalance in any one of these three areas can affect the health and balance of the other areas.

For most of recorded history (and, I imagine, through prerecorded history as well) the notion that we are an integrated whole was accepted unquestioningly. The religious tribal leader—priest or shaman—was also the tribal medicine man. Physical illness was seen as emanating from a mental or spiritual source, while spiritual states were often induced by the ingestion of herbs or other substances. Hippocrates was teaching healers to care for the whole person some 2,500 years ago.

Over time, however, the Western model dichotomizing the mind and body began to prevail. Louis Pasteur introduced the concept of the germ and removed a great deal of mystery and myth from illness. Western medicine placed increasing emphasis on the body as the repository of all answers to illness.

Physicians also became more and more specialized. The old-fashioned kindly family doctor with his black bag was replaced by specialists of all varieties. Specialization is for the most part a good thing. It enables doctors to become highly adept and proficient in a given field and to develop expertise that in today's rapidly changing world of medicine and medical technology would be impossible for the generalist.

However, the downside of specialization has been that often we forget that the body works as a single organic unit. An imbalance in one system can be caused by an imbalance in another system and can, in turn, cause an imbalance in yet a third system. As we will see when we take a closer look at cervical disease, an imbalance in the digestive system can, in turn, cause an imbalance in the reproductive hormonal system, which can, in turn, make it more difficult for the body to resist the destructive impact of infection with HPV. So while the primary actors in the HPV drama may be the genital tract and cervix, we cannot ignore the other players, such as the liver and the gut.

The patient's spiritual and emotional state also cannot be ignored. Holistic medicine addresses the whole person—mind, body, *and* spirit. Examining all aspects of the person means that we are not only attending to symptoms of illness, but also to the causes of the illness—mental and spiritual as well as physical. Neglecting causes and treating only the symptoms is like bailing water out of a leaky boat without plugging the leak. You might get rid of all the water at the bottom of the boat but unless the fundamental source of the problem— the hole in the boat—is fixed, the boat will continue to leak.

When I work with patients, I tell them to view their illness as an opportunity to heal not only the particular situation at hand, but also the broader imbalances that might be present. Illness can be used as a vehicle to create balance.

Balance is the key word here. When all systems are in a state of balance, we feel most fully alive. The primary objective of holistic medicine is to help patients attain that state—a condition of optimum physical, environmental, mental, emotional, spiritual, and social health. And, even more important, to do so with an attitude of respect and unconditional love toward themselves.

EFFECTS OF THE LIVER AND GASTROINTESTINAL TRACT ON CERVICAL HEALTH

In Chapter 4, you learned that although 60 to 80 percent of Americans are infected with HPV, only a small percentage will go on to develop symptoms such as cervical dysplasia, cervical cancer, or genital warts. When you are in optimal health, your body is better able to fight off the damaging effects of HPV and prevent it from wreaking havoc on your genital tract. Optimal health is creatied by a state of balance among several organs and systems. Let's look at some of these organs and systems that have an impact on your cervical and genital health.

THE LIVER AND ITS IMPACT ON HORMONES

We begin with one of the most fascinating, multifaceted and complex organs—the liver. Located in the upper right quadrant of your abdomen, the liver is responsible for an enormous number of tasks. It converts the sugar and starch you eat into a form that your body can use—either for storage or for immediate energy. It plays an important role in detoxifying your system—converting potentially toxic substances into innocuous forms so that they can be excreted safely.

The liver is particularly important in maintaining correct hormonal balance. Your reproductive organs produce several sex hormones that work together to maintain optimal reproductive health. These include estrogen, progesterone, testosterone, and DHEA. Additionally, your adrenal glands produce DHEA and cortisol, which are involved in regulating your response to stress. If you have too much or too little of any of these hormones, you will experience unpleasant or even dangerous symptoms. Too much testosterone, for example, may make you excessively masculine. You may develop facial hair and your voice may deepen. But too little testosterone may cause you to feel fatigue and lack of sexual desire.

One of the most important balances to maintain is between estrogen and progesterone. Each hormone serves a different function. Estrogen promotes sexual maturation, stimulates ovulation, is responsible for preparing the breast tissue for lactation when you are nursing a baby, and is responsible for the first phase of your menstrual cycle—the release of the egg from the ovary. Estrogen also has an impact on your health that goes beyond your reproductive functions—it promotes cardiovascular health, skin elasticity, bone density, and vaginal moisture and suppleness.

Progesterone keeps the estrogen in tow and modulates estrogen levels. It is responsible for the second phase of the menstrual cycle by causing the excessive uterine lining to be shed during menstruation. It is also necessary for fertility. Additionally, progesterone regulates fluid balance and has a generally calming effect.

For the body to function optimally, estrogen and progesterone must be properly balanced. When estrogen levels are too high, a condition called *estrogen dominance* occurs. This condition has been associated with a variety of conditions, including cervical dysplasia. Let's take a closer look at how that works—and particularly at the role of the liver.

It is the job of the liver to take circulating estrogen—specifically estrone and estradiol, which are two types of estrogen—and convert it into a form that can be excreted by the body. The liver performs this function in two phases. Phase I converts the estrogens into water-soluble intermediary substances and Phase II combines them with other substances so that they become water-soluble and ready for excretion.

During Phase I, the estrogens are formed into one of three intermediary substances: 2-hydroxyestrone; 4-hydroxyestrone or 16-alphahydroxyestrone. Of these three substances, the safest and most desirable is 2-hydroxyestrone. Numbers 4 and 16 have been associated with the overproduction of *quinones*—carcinogenic substances that we'll return to below. The 16-alphahydroxyesterone has been implicated in all diseases of estrogen dominance, from cervical dysplasia to breast cancer.

Phase II takes the hydroxyestrogens through the *methylation, glucoronidation* or *sulfation pathways*. These are a series of chemical changes that combine the estrogen metabolites resulting from Phase I with a substance such as methyl, sulfur or an amino acid group. They are then ready for excretion through the intestines or the kidney.

What can go wrong with these systems? Plenty, because they are so complex and delicately balanced. A malfunction at the Phase I level can cause an overproduction of the destructive 4- and 16-hydroxyestrogens. And a malfunction at the Phase II level can cause these destructive estrogen metabolites to remain within the system rather than being excreted. Keep these phases in mind because we will return to them when we discuss nutrition.

GUT FEELINGS—A DIALOGUE BETWEEN YOUR LIVER AND YOUR STOMACH

We all know that our gastrointestinal tract—our gut—is responsible for the absorption of nutrients from food and for the production of waste. Most of us don't realize, however, just how amazing and complex the process is—and how easily it can go wrong in subtle ways. I stress the word *subtle* because we all know how it feels when our stomach is really out of sorts—most of us have at one time or another suffered from a twenty-four-hour stomach virus or intestinal flu, and we know how miserable that is. But even when we're feeling fine and our stomachs appear to be behaving themselves, we can still be suffering from imbalances in what is called the *intestinal flora*. We can be deficient in the "good" bacteria that participate in digesting our food and allowing maximum absorption of nutrients.

Having very low levels of "good" bacteria leads to an overgrowth of "bad" bacteria with nothing to counteract their negative impact. We call that a state of *gut* or *intestinal dysbiosis*. Gut dysbiosis can be caused by a poor diet. It can also be caused by taking antibiotics that destroy not only the "bad" bacteria they're designed to fight, but also the good, healthy bacteria in your intestines. For this reason, it is important to replace those missing intestinal bacteria with *probiotic supplementation*. Eating yogurt, which contains live cultures, or taking acidophilus or bifidobacteria supplements can accomplish this.

One of the destructive effects of gut dysbiosis is that when the liver sends the estrogen that's been prepared and packaged for excretion through the bile duct and into the intestine, the bad bacteria begin to break down and "unpackage" the estrogen, undoing all the liver's hard work. The enzyme responsible for unpackaging estradiol is *beta-glucuronidase*—an enzyme that forces apart the glucuronic acid molecule from the estrogen, sending the estrogen back into circulation. This enzyme is produced by "bad" intestinal bacteria.

Now the liver is really overwhelmed. It is confronted with the very same estrogens it just finished processing—plus new estrogens it must take care of. The overtaxed liver not only works harder, but also depletes the available nutrients necessary for Phase I and Phase II to be enacted successfully. Needless to say, an exhausted liver will, over time, become less effective at performing its necessary tasks, including the processing and excretion of estrogen. Therefore, estrogen levels will rise beyond what is healthy; the stronger and potentially carcinogenic 16- and 4-hydroxyestrogens will increase; and the condition of estrogen dominance ensues.

HOW DO I KNOW IF MY LIVER IS WORKING?

Before we discuss what happens in the body during estrogen dominance and how it can increase the chances of cervical dysplasia, I'd like to take a moment to preempt a question you might have about the liver.

If you go to your doctor and undergo a standard liver profile test, the cells within your liver cells will be measured. These enzymes are called *hepatocytes*. The findings your physician receives will reflect only the most major disruption and breakdown of these cells. If your liver is severely damaged—let's say you have hepatitis, for example—the extreme breakdown will be reflected on this type of test. However, more subtle changes will not show up. The liver profile measures only the most drastic changes. The liver cells may not be breaking down, but this doesn't mean that they're working well.

To evaluate more subtle changes in the liver, I usually order a *functional liver test*. This test challenges the liver with substances known to place stress on liver function, such as caffeine, acetaminophen, or aspirin. A normal liver should be able to process and handle these substances efficiently, despite the extra output of energy and liver enzymes necessary. A dysfunctional liver won't be able to do that. The functional liver test measures liver metabolites during Phase I and Phase II. This gives a clear indication of how the liver is actually functioning.

ESTROGEN DOMINANCE AND CERVICAL DYSPLASIA

For hormones to be effective, they can't just circulate around the body in a free-floating fashion. They must be "received" by an organ so they can be put to work. You have all kinds of different hormone receptors throughout your body. They function like beckoning fingers, each with its own shape and design. When the appropriate hormone drifts by, the receptor "grabs" and holds on to it.

The cervix has many estrogen receptors. The presence of excessive free-floating estrogen in the body means that too much will be deposited in the cervix. This is problematic because estrogen is a growth hormone. Just as it stimulates the uterus to pile on extra levels of tissue during the first phase of your menstrual cycle, so it stimulates tissue growth in other areas as well. Excessive cervical growth translates into abnormal cell development and cervical dysplasia.

Moreover, the excessive estrogen levels overwhelm the liver, as we discussed above. The liver begins malfunctioning. It produces too many 4- and 16-hydroxyestrogens, which go on to become compounds called quinones. These quinones have been associated with cancer in many regions of the body, including the cervix. Scientists are still studying the mechanism through which quinones attack the DNA in cells, inhibiting the normal process of cell death and causing the cells to proliferate. As you know from Chapters 3 and 4, this process of uncontrolled cell growth is cancer.

While all the pieces of the quinone-cancer puzzle are still in the process of being assembled, scientists are pretty sure that the process through which 4-hydroxyestrogens are converted into quinones is *oxidation*—or the adding of oxygen. We generally think of oxygen as a good thing—and indeed it is. Oxygen is essential to life. However, oxygen in the wrong place and time can be destructive. Think of what happens when iron oxidizes as a result of water damage. Rust forms and eventually erodes the iron. Many conditions including aging and degenerative diseases are associated with the negative effects of oxidation. We will return to this when we discuss antioxidants, which are nutrients that can prevent or interrupt the oxidation process.

Oxidation plays a role in the way quinones cause DNA breakdown. Quinones are strong oxidants. They are called *free radicals*. No, this is not some term borrowed from the political climate of the 1960s. Free radicals are chemicals that roam the body, causing oxidative damage. When quinones combine with a DNA molecule, they pull an electron off the DNA and oxidize it. The damaged DNA if not adequately repaired can go on to turn the cell into a cancer factory.

I hope that this journey through the liver and gut has given you a more thorough understanding of the myriad factors involved in maintaining good health in general and good cervical health in particular, and how dysfunctions in these areas can lead to compromised health. Understanding how these systems work will help you learn what nutritional factors contribute to the difference between being infected with HPV but fighting it off so that you don't develop any symptoms, versus coming down with a case of cervical disease or genital warts.

A Healthier Liver, A Healthier Cervix

NUTRITION AND LIVER FUNCTION

Like every other organ in the body, the liver must be fed appropriate nutrients in order to function optimally. The most important nutrients for the liver are folic acid, vitamins B_6, B_3, and vitamin B_{12}; zinc; magnesium; and S-adenosyl methionine (SAM-e). All of these are important for the methylation, gluconidation, and sulfation pathways. If you are deficient in these nutrients, your liver will be unable to carry out Phase I effectively, and too many 4- and 16-hydroxyestrogens may be formed, rather than the beneficial 2s. And if Phase II cannot be enacted properly, the hydroxyestrogens will not be packaged for excretion and will remain in your body also helping to set up the "estrogen dominant" state.

Now let's look at the next phase of the process, Phase II. If you are not eating a diet rich in antioxidants, the quinones will attack your DNA, using the process of oxidation. Carotenes, vitamins C and E, selenium, green tea, and the spice turmeric all contain antioxidants. Some of the chemical compounds that have antioxidant properties are flavonoids, bioflavonoids, isoflavones, and lignans.

The average American diet is woefully deficient in these antioxidants. I like to call it SAD—the Standard American Diet. High in animal protein and fat and low in fiber, vegetables, and fruits, SAD contributes to an array of negative health conditions, including cardiovascular disease, degenerative diseases such as Alzheimer's, arthritis, and cancer. Study after study has found a strong association between a diet rich in vegetables, soy, and fiber and a lower incidence of cancer. That's because these beneficial nutrients are found in vegetables. The more vegetables you eat—preferably spanning the full range of colors—the more of these nutrients you consume. In particular, vegetables of the *Brassica* family, also known as the cruciferous vegetables, including broccoli, Brussels sprouts, and cabbage, contain an important substance called indole-3-carbinol (I3C). I3C helps the liver make more of the beneficial 2-hydroxyestrogen and less of the damaging 4- and 16-hydroxyestrogens. As you learned in Chapter 9, this important substance is being studied for the treatment of respiratory papillomatosis. Its effects are quite powerful and far-reaching. It has also been studied for its positive effects in cases of cervical dysplasia. Nine women with cervical dysplasia who were given a twelve-week course of I3C supplementation were compared to nine women who received a placebo. Those who received the supplement showed great improvement at the end of the study, while those who received the placebo were unchanged. So when Grandma told you to eat your broccoli, it seems that she was right!

While vegetables should form the foundation of your diet, there are many other foods that supply antioxidants. Soy and kudzu contain beneficial flavonoids and bioflavonoids. Flaxseeds contain lignans. And all vegetables and whole grains contain fiber.

Why is fiber important? It not only helps avoid the discomfort and inconvenience of irregular bowel movements, but it also helps avoid the medical damage caused by constipation. When there is a buildup of waste matter in the intestinal tract, there is an increase of the "bad" bacteria we discussed earlier. This buildup can be caused not only by constipation but also by inefficient intestinal housecleaning. Fiber doesn't only serve to move fecal material along but also serves as a broom or scrubbing brush for your intestinal walls. Imagine how your floor would look if it were never swept or scrubbed! This is how your intestines look if you don't eat enough fiber. A low-fiber diet is heavily implicated in the buildup of *pathogenic,* or illness-causing bacteria present when there is gut dysbiosis. As we discussed, this condition leads to the unpackaging of estrogens that are ready to be excreted. Their reentry into the body causes estrogen dominance and its related problems.

One of the best protections you have against cancer is to eat a diet rich in soy products, kudzu, flaxseeds, whole grains, and the full gamut of fruits and vegetables. However, diet isn't always enough. The growing conditions of produce in this country are often not conducive to the development of maximum nutritional content. And to attain these nutrients to counteract some of the negative effects of other aspects of the American lifestyle—such as the damaging impact of pesticides, fuels, and plastics—we would have to eat far more than is desirable or even healthy. For this reason, I recommend nutritional supplementation. (See pages 130 and 135 for specific recommendations.)

REDUCING STRESS

A high-stress lifestyle places great strain on the entire body and has been associated with all kinds of damaging effects—including cervical dysplasia. Stress increases the production of cortisol and adrenaline, which are hormones secreted by your adrenal glands. Sometime during prehistory, the adrenal glands of our ancestors developed this highly adaptive mechanism to help combat the stressors of the jungle— storms, charging bears, floods, and the like. During life-threatening crises, the adrenal glands poured out their hormones that energized the body, enabling the individual to engage in the "fight-or-flight" response—to either combat the menacing force, or to successfully run away from it.

Our ancestors faced stressors that came and went quickly. In today's world, however, our stressors usually aren't wild animals or natural disasters but are overdrawn bank statements, recalcitrant teenagers, nagging bosses, or delayed subway trains. We are also stressed by deeper forces, such as the gnawing unhappiness we feel in an inappropriate employment situation or unsatisfying marriage, the deleterious effects of abuse, or the daily strain of financial and scheduling demands. While the hormones produced by our adrenal glands might have been ideal for the jungle, they are inappropriate for the city or the suburbs. They prepare the body for an intense output of physical activity that never takes place. The high levels of cortisol and adrenaline increase insulin levels so that more stored carbohydrate can be rapidly converted into energy. But the increased insulin also leads to increased estrogen in the body. Here's how it works:

When hormones circulate through your body, they are usually bound to other chemicals that prevent them from latching on to any available receptor. In fact, 90 percent of the hormones in your body circulate in a bound form. There is a special substance, a protein called *globulin* that's responsible for binding to estrogen and making sure that only a small amount of free and available estrogen is circulating at any given time.

Insulin tends to decrease this sex hormone–binding globulin. When insulin levels are dramatically and repeatedly elevated by overproduction of cortisol and adrenaline, globulin levels are dramatically and repeatedly diminished. More and more free estrogen is allowed to roam and leap onto beckoning and available receptors. While appropriate amounts of sex hormones, like estrogen, are needed for normal functioning, excessive amounts that are unbound can create an imbalance of hormones leading to all the problems associated with estrogen dominance.

Elevated levels of insulin also overtax the liver. Remember that the liver is responsible for converting stored sugar into a form that becomes energy. The liver is working very hard to do this. Now additional loads of estrogen are dumped at its doorstep—at the very time it is busy concentrating on something else. These new loads of estrogen cannot be effectively processed. As we discussed earlier, they become 4- and 16-hydroxyestrogens, then quinones that find their way to sensitive areas such as the cervix and begin the assault on the DNA that ultimately can lead to cancer.

Stress reduction, then, is not a luxury. It's not a frill. It is an integral part of any healing program. And it's a process that involves all aspects of your life—your environment, relationships, attitudes, and beliefs, as well as your spiritual practices. For example, creating a lower-stress lifestyle is valuable and important, but won't do much good if you are anxious and worried about your "idleness" or spin your internal wheels about some other issue. Cognitive approaches, such as insight-oriented psychotherapy, are extremely helpful, but often aren't enough to bring about the deeper internal changes that are necessary for true relaxation, self-acceptance, and a sense of well-being and wholeness. For this reason, I usually recommend an array of approaches in addition to conventional psychotherapy. These include hypnosis, guided imagery, visualization, and specific stress-reduction techniques such as meditation, yoga, qi gong, and tai chi. Hands-on contact with a healer through such mediums as Reiki, therapeutic touch, and massage can also be powerful stress reducers.

Now that we've looked at physical and emotional contributors to cervical disorders, let's look at holistic approaches to treating the disorders.

UNCONDITIONAL LOVE AS A HEALING TOOL

As a physician, I believe that unconditional love is my most powerful healing tool. I find that optimal healing occurs in an environment of unconditional love. But unconditional love can't be confined only to my office. We are a society in which all too many people dislike themselves. The spiritual leader of the Tibetan people, the Dalai Lama, has been quoted as expressing surprise and distress at the existence and extent of self-hatred in prosperous Western countries such as our own. This was a phenomenon quite new to him. I encourage you to begin your healing journey in the spirit of love for yourself. By self-love, I don't mean self-indulgence, narcissism, or greed at the expense of others. Rather, I mean a deep compassion for yourself, gentleness toward your flaws and foibles—none of us is perfect, and we all have flaws and foibles—and a love for yourself as a spirit, a child of the Universe. This type of self-embrace brings a profound calm and can be more healing than any drug or herb. It is an attitude that will deepen as you continue on your healing journey and will spill over to the others in your life.

WHEN YOUR PAP SMEAR IS ABNORMAL

ASCUS AND LGSIL: PROACTIVE WATCHING AND WAITING

By now you know that ASCUS is the most confusing result you can get on a Pap smear. If this result comes back from the lab, I order an HPV typing test. This provides me with valuable information regarding the possible presence of HPV and the strain of virus. If your test results are negative for the presence of the virus, then I am comfortable with a watch-and-wait protocol and conduct a repeat Pap smear in about three months. If HPV is present, I immediately perform a colposcopy and biopsy to determine whether there is a lesion. If the results point to LGSIL, I feel I am safe in recommending to "watch and wait."

I believe a conservative approach is possible even though LGSIL indicates the presence of a low-grade lesion and even if the lesion is caused by a high-grade HPV strain. Many low-grade lesions do reverse themselves without intervention. Studies have shown that chance of mild cervical dysplasia self-reversing are between 1 and 2 percent, perhaps as high as 5 percent. But if the patient takes nutritional supplements and antioxidants, there is a 20 to 25 percent reversion rate.

During the watching and waiting, however, I do more than simply take a passive, hands-folded spectator approach. I prescribe an aggressive regimen of natural treatments designed to strengthen the body's ability to fight the virus and reverse the symptoms while still at an early stage.

NUTRITIONAL INTAKE AND SUPPLEMENTATION

I urge patients to eat foods rich in folic acid. These include dark leafy vegetables, broccoli, lima beans, citrus fruit, soybeans, and black-eyed peas. I also prescribe a basic multivitamin-multimineral supplement in addition to daily doses of 10 milligrams of folic acid, 3,000 to 4,000 milligrams of vitamin C, 50,000 IU of beta-carotene, 30 milligrams of zinc, and 400 micrograms of selenium.

VAGINAL NUTRITIONAL SUPPOSITORIES

Vitamin A is an anti-inflammatory nutrient that supports the lining cells all over the body, including the lining of the cervix, and is excellent at repairing mucous membranes. Used in suppository form, its repair properties can go to work directly on the affected site. Vag-Pak suppositories consist of vitamin A, magnesium sulfate, and glycerin, which all have anti-inflammatory properties. Additionally, they contain tea tree oil and an herb called thuja. Tea tree is a commonly used herb for a variety of dermatological conditions, and thuja has antiviral properties.

Vitamin C is a powerful antioxidant. It will counteract the oxidative effects of the excessive quinones we discussed earlier. Herbal-C suppositories contain additional herbs, such as echinacea, which strengthen the immune system.

When HPV is diagnosed, I recommend the Papillo suppository, which contains vitamin A and thuja oil, as well as other antiviral herbs, instead of the Herbal-C suppositories.

When the HPV test is negative, I recommend two series of suppositories used on alternating weeks:

- Week 1: Vitamin A suppositories daily for six days, and Vag-Pak suppositories on the seventh day.
- Week 2: Herbal-C suppositories daily for six days, and Vag-Pak suppositories on the seventh day.

All of these suppositories are available by mail order. See the Resources section for more information on purchasing them.

LIFESTYLE CHANGES

I urge my patients to look at and modify aspects of their lifestyle that are known to contribute to cervical dysplasia. These include drugs and alcohol, which take a toll on the entire system, and smoking, which intensifies Phase I, creating more hydroxyestrogen metabolites that are too numerous to be adequately handled during Phase II. We also know that the by-products of nicotine are concentrated a thousand times in the cervical tissue. Birth control pills are known to cause nutritional deficiencies in folic acid, the other B vitamins, magnesium, and zinc. Many studies have linked the use of oral contraceptives with cervical dysplasia and cancer. Together with the patient, I work out alternative forms of contraception. I also recommend that my patients alter their nutritional intake by increasing consumption of vegetables, fruits, whole grains, and soy products while decreasing their consumption of refined flour and sugar (which stress the liver), animal-based protein, and saturated fat.

As mentioned earlier, one of the most important aspects of lifestyle modification is stress reduction. I discuss with my patients the areas of stress and conflict in their lives. We examine the many stress-reduction techniques and decide which might be most appropriate. While psychotherapy might be extremely useful for one person, it might be less effective for another. Some people respond well to sedentary techniques, such as meditation and hypnosis, while others prefer more active meditational practices, such as yoga or qi gong. The visually inclined may find guided imagery and visualization to be powerful healing tools. Body scan meditation, a meditative technique taught by Jon Kabat-Zinn in his book *Full Catastrophe Living,* is a powerful exercise to help reverse cervical dysplasia. Those who are more auditory in focus may prefer a talk-based or musical therapeutic approach. Whatever works to reduce your stress will be helpful and should be initiated during this heal-and-wait period. I prefer that terminology to "watch and wait" because it implies an active process of healing during the waiting period.

REPEAT PAP SMEAR

In the case of ASCUS without HPV, I repeat the Pap smear after two or three months. If it is normal, my patient can discontinue the suppositories, but should continue taking a basic multivitamin and lower doses of folic acid and the other antioxidants. She should also continue to follow a balanced nutritional program. These are essential health maintenance tools for life and for continuing to keep HPV at bay. I also suggest continuing any stress reduction techniques for as long as necessary.

In the case of LGSIL, I repeat the colposcopy as well as the Pap smear. Even if the colposcopy and Pap smear are normal, I follow the patient closely. I repeat the Pap smear after another four-month period, then at four-month intervals for one year. Then if the Pap smears are normal, I perform Pap smears biannually thereafter. Once there is a diagnosis of high-risk HPV, I recommend that the antioxidants and folic acid be taken for life. The dosages may be decreased with time as long as the Pap smears stay normal.

I encourage my patients to regard ASCUS and LGSIL as "wake-up calls" from their bodies. These are red flags the body is waving, signaling the presence of imbalances and unresolved issues—physical, emotional, or spiritual—that need addressing. I urge them to see this distressing diagnosis as a gift rather than a curse and to use it as a way to heal not only the cervix but other areas of their lives as well.

TREATMENT OF HGSIL

There's much less room for experimentation and conservative waiting when it comes to HGSIL. These lesions can easily progress to become invasive cancer. It's likely that it's a high-risk strain of HPV that's causing the lesion. When HGSIL is diagnosed, I recommend the LEEP procedure or a cold-knife cone biopsy after performing a colposcopy to be sure that there is no invasive cancer present. And if cancer is present, I recommend surgical removal of the cervix. Conventionally this is done by hysterectomy.

However, this doesn't mean that HGSIL cannot be approached holistically. Like ASCUS and LGSIL, it is a wake-up call—only it's more urgent. The extent of damage is an indicator of the extent of imbalance and the issues that need addressing and healing.

When possible, and especially if my patient wishes to become pregnant at some point, I recommend the most conservative surgical procedure available. After a surgical procedure, I recommend vitamin A applied topically to hasten healing. Castor oil hot packs—castor oil wrapped in flannel and heated with a source such as a heating pad—is soothing when applied to the pelvic area. Originally recommended by the twentieth-century mystic Edgar Cayce, these hot packs work by stimulating the immune system, helping with lymph drainage, and reducing toxins. They hasten the healing of inflammation, and when applied to the abdomen over the liver, they seem to boost liver function.

Of course, the vitamins, nutritional supplements, and mind-body techniques that I recommend for ASCUS and LGSIL are equally important for HGSIL. They assist the body in fighting not only the HPV but also other potentially carcinogenic processes. These nutrients require lifelong supplementation.

TREATMENT OF INVASIVE CANCER

As with HGSIL, there is no time to wait or experiment when a cancerous lesion has penetrated the basement membrane and invaded the surrounding areas. As discussed in Chapter 7, you might require one of many possible surgical procedures. And beyond surgery, you might require chemotherapy or radiation.

A complete and exhaustive discussion of holistic approaches to cancer is well beyond the purview of a single chapter. Indeed, tomes could be devoted to this rapidly expanding field. If you go to the bookstore or search the Internet, you will find hundreds if not thousands of books, articles, and Web sites dedicated to complementary approaches to cancer. An overwhelming and bewildering array of options will present themselves, and it may be difficult for you to sort out the wheat from the chaff or the quacks and charlatans from the authentic healers. Toward the end of this book, you will find suggestions for further reading as well as a list of several reliable, legitimate, and helpful resources. This section will provide you with some basic modalities to get you started.

ACUPUNCTURE

Acupuncture is an ancient, well-respected Chinese healing technique that can be used together with conventional cancer therapy. In acupuncture, tiny needles are inserted into the skin at key points to assist the body in redressing imbalances in the flow of energy. According to traditional Chinese medicine, illness is caused when the normal flow of energy through the system is disrupted. Western scientists who have studied acupuncture have arrived at different explanations for its effectiveness—for example, it is believed that, for reasons that remain unclear, acupuncture stimulates endorphins in the brain. These are the brain's "feel-good" chemicals that help stabilize our moods and also help reduce pain when we are injured.

Whatever the reason for its success, the National Institutes of Health (NIH) has endorsed acupuncture for its effectiveness in reducing pain and also combating the nausea and other unpleasant symptoms commonly associated with chemotherapy. Other methods of deep bodywork, including acupressure, can also be effective and might be useful if you are needle-shy.

PHYTOTHERAPY

Phytotherapy, or plant-based therapy, can be used for a variety of purposes. Some herbs can reduce the toxic impact and negative side effects of chemotherapy and radiation. In fact, there are herbs that can even increase sensitivity to these treatments, thereby rendering them more effective. Other herbs work by strengthening the immune system. This helps the body fight the cancer and also combat infection that can attack while the body is vulnerable and weakened by chemotherapy or radiation. Some herbs improve blood flow to the affected tissues and assist the lymph nodes in clearing the system, some are anti-inflammatory, while still others assist the liver in the detoxification process. We previously discussed antioxidant vitamins, but there are antioxidant herbs as well. These can also be helpful in combating free radicals and their oxidative damage. Dealing with cancer places great strain on the emotions and is one of the most stressful experiences anyone can face. Fortunately, there are herbs that can help reduce stress.

I hope that this brief glance at phytotherapy will help you understand that there are numerous useful adjuncts to conventional cancer therapies that can be comforting on a short-term level, and may even speed the healing process. There are many herbs that may be helpful in your healing. I advise you to work with a health-care practitioner who is familiar with these substances to personalize an herbal regimen that addresses your own individual needs.

Astragalus

Astragalus (*Astragalus membranoceus*) is a useful adjunct to chemotherapy and radiation. It helps stop debilitating sweating, expels toxins, and helps combat fatigue. It also has general immune-strengthening properties.

Dandelion Root

While it's true that dandelions (*Taraxacum radix*) are pretty yellow weeds, their roots have been traditionally used for healing purposes. Dandelion is an herb that helps the liver in the detoxification process. It also has laxative properties.

Dong Quai

Dong Quai (*Angelica sinesis*) has been used in traditional Chinese medicine for more than 2,000 years and specifically works on the female reproductive system. Used traditionally to regulate the menstrual cycle, it also serves to keep blood moving efficiently. Traditionally, dong quai is used in combination with other herbs.

Echinacea

Echinacea (*Echinacea angustifolia* and *purpurea*) is one of the most commonly used and widely studied herbs. It stimulates the immune system and thereby enhances resistance to viral and bacterial infections.

Ginseng

Ginseng (*Panax ginseng*) is an ancient herb classically used to strengthen adrenal function and assist the adrenal glands in the production of stress hormones. It is an *adaptogen,* meaning that it helps the body to adapt to a variety of stressors, including chemotherapy, radiation, and emotional stress. It decreases the side effects of some chemotherapy drugs. In addition, it may assist the body in the process of cellular differentiation, which plays such a crucial role in the transformation zone and the development of cervical disease.

Grape Seed Extract

Grape seed extract, or Pycnogenol, is a very potent bioflavonoid that works in conjunction with vitamin C to help strengthen capillary walls, reduce inflammation, and help prevent cancer.

Kava

Kava (*Piper methysticum*) is a calming herb used for anxiety. Again, anxiety is a normal response to a life-threatening illness, and can also be the side effect of some chemotherapeutic agents. Kava induces a mild feeling of euphoria and is very soothing.

Milk Thistle

Milk thistle (*Silybum marianum*) is an antioxidant known for its protective and restorative effects on the liver.

Pau d'Arco

Pau d'arco (*Tabebuia avellanedae*) is taken from the inner bark of the Tabebuia tree, which is native to the Caribbean region. It has been used for treatment of colds and other infections. Some studies have also found it to be effective in treating cancer. Certainly it is known to enhance immune function.

Rehmannia

Rehmannia (*Rehmannia glutinosa*) is an ancient Chinese herb, traditionally used as a tonic. It has an anti-inflammatory effect and helps with fevers and conditions caused by deficiencies in body fluids, such as night sweats, dry mouth or throat, and constipation.

St. John's Wort

Often called "Nature's Prozac," St. John's wort (*Hypericum perforatum*) has been widely studied for its antidepressant effects and can be useful in combating the emotional "downs" associated with cancer—both those caused by the psychological issues raised by the disease itself and those caused by the impact of chemotherapy.

Shiitake and Reishi Mushrooms

Japanese studies suggest that substances present in shiitake and reishi mushrooms (*Lentinula edodes* and *Ganoderma lucidum*) stimulate immune function and the synthesis of interferon molecules—small proteins with antiviral effects produced by the body.

Siberian Ginseng

Siberian ginseng (*Eleutherococcus senticosus*) is not actually ginseng at all, although it performs some similar functions. Like ginseng, it is an adaptogen. It also improves healing and reduces side effects from chemotherapy, radiation, and surgery.

Turmeric

Turmeric (*Curcuma longa*) is an antioxidant that appears to inhibit the oxidation of fats in the liver.

Withania

This herb (*Withania somnifera*) is indigenous to India and has been brought to the West via the Indian herbal tradition, which is called Ayurveda. Like ginseng, it is an adaptogen. It is most useful in dealing with the weight loss that often accompanies cancer or that results from cancer therapies.

PSYCHOLOGICAL/SPIRITUAL SUPPORT

Once again, I can't emphasize enough the role that stress reduction and emotional/spiritual healing play in handling cancer. Attending a support group for cancer patients, participating in individual psychotherapy, and finding a spiritual network or environment that is consistent with your beliefs and worldview are all emotionally comforting and can also have important practical ramifications. Others who are familiar with the stages and pitfalls of cancer treatment can assist you in finding solutions to common problems and can provide you with moral support. Mind/body techniques such as those discussed above can help you do the deeper work and resolve some of the less-accessible emotional and spiritual issues that arise.

Please note that by "spiritual" I don't necessarily mean that you need to adhere to an established religious system or adopt any special dogma. Rather, your spirit needs to be nurtured by whatever feels correct to you. For some people, a walk along the beach, a hike through the woods, or watching a beautiful sunset can provide a connection with nature and can be a spiritual experience. For others, the exhilarating "runner's high" following a good jog can serve the purpose. Still others feel a deep, almost mystical connection to art, music, or gardening. I encourage you to find and engage in regular activities that are not only relaxing (a movie or television sitcom can also be relaxing) but also address the deeper, spiritual dimensions.

Once, cancer was considered a certain death sentence. With today's more sophisticated conventional techniques, there is hope. Many individuals with cancer *do* achieve permanent remission. Taking a holistic approach increases your chances of survival dramatically. Equally important, a holistic approach enables you to turn the illness into an opportunity for growth and healing on all levels, and to build your reserves so that the illness does not recur.

TREATMENT FOR GENITAL WARTS

The first step in treating genital warts is removing them. Once the warts have been removed, the challenge becomes preventing them from recurring. Patients with genital warts should follow the same nutritional and supplement regimen that I prescribe for patients with cervical dysplasia. I also recommend the immune-strengthening herbs outlined in the section on the treatment of cancer. These assist the body in fighting the virus so that it doesn't manifest itself again.

ADDRESSING HPV IN MEN AND CHILDREN

The nutritional recommendations that help women to fight off the disease are also helpful for men who may be carrying the virus. Particularly if you have the virus, your partner should follow such a regimen to help fight it. Your partner's liver needs the same nutrients yours does for optimal function. Smoking, substance abuse, and multiple sex partners place men at increased risk of manifesting HPV, as do the unhealthy aspects of the American lifestyle—particularly the "SAD" diet and high-stress mode of living. Eating nutritiously and engaging in the same stress-reduction techniques I recommended above will be as helpful for men as for women.

While it is possible to bring HPV levels below clinically measurable quantities, the virus probably can't ever be totally eradicated from the system once you have been infected. However, you can prevent it from manifesting itself as genital warts or cervical disease by instituting healthy lifestyle changes, including eating an optimal diet; taking vitamin/mineral supplements; quitting smoking, alcohol, and drugs; exercising; and eliminating stress.

I wish you healing, good health, and inner peace.

CARLA'S STORY

Carla was understandably distressed when I called to tell her that she had a slightly abnormal Pap smear. "Do I have cancer?" she asked anxiously. I explained that her diagnosis was ASCUS—atypical squamous cells of undetermined significance. "Your test results say that you may have a dysplastic process going on—this means that your cells may be changing in precancerous ways, rather than just reacting to infection or hormonal changes. But we don't know that for sure." I told her I would order an HPV test. "This will give us more information."

"HPV?" she asked. "What's that? I've never heard of it."

I told her about the human papilloma virus and its role in cervical cancer. "If your HPV test is negative, we can be fairly sure you don't have a cancerous process going on. But if it's positive, and you have a high-risk strain, we may have to be more aggressive because these strains are associated with cervical cancer."

Carla was even more upset when her HPV test was positive for a high-risk viral strain. After a nasty divorce and six tumultuous years of unhappy relationships, she had just started dating someone new and felt that this relationship might be "the one" for her. "My life is just getting on track, and now this is coming along to ruin it," she moaned.

Upon further questioning, I learned that her notion of a "life on track" left much to be desired. A thirty-eight-year-old attorney with a high-stress job, she smoked a pack of cigarettes a day. Her long working hours prevented her from exercising regularly or eating well. Breakfast consisted of coffee and a bagel. Lunch was a tuna fish salad on white bread, and her idea of a vegetable was the limp carrot or celery in her Chinese take-out dinner. She had been taking oral contraceptives for many years.

We scheduled an immediate colposcopy and were very relieved when the biopsy results showed only a low-grade dysplastic lesion. Carla and I discussed the significance of this finding and decided that we would not go further to perform a cone biopsy of her cervix, because she wanted to have children in the future. Instead, we agreed on a regimen of vitamins and supplements, including folic acid, mixed carotenes, vitamin C, zinc, and selenium. She would also use vaginal suppositories for three months.

Carla agreed to stop smoking and discontinue her use of the birth control pill. We did some problem-solving around matters of food and exercise, and she agreed to start eating more regular and nutritious meals. She also decided to join a gym and start exercising regularly.

Carla's conversations with me and the disturbing Pap smear results were an alert about unresolved emotional issues, not just physical ones. She realized that, pleased as she was with her new boyfriend, the loose ends and unhealed self-doubt left from her marriage could damage her new relationship. Without prodding or pushing from me, she entered psychotherapy to explore and resolve problems from the earlier relationship, and from the unhappy liaisons of the intervening six years.

Three months later, when we repeated the colposcopy and biopsies, we were both thrilled to find that the cells were normal. Carla's lifestyle changes and her commitment to the holistic program had led to this gratifying reversal. Although she realized that she would probably remain HPV-positive for the rest of her life, she understood that she could have some control over how the virus expressed itself; by maintaining optimal health she could prevent a recurrence.

11

How You Can Win the War Against HPV

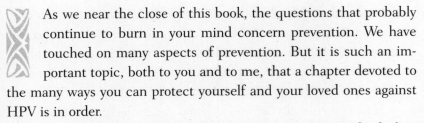 As we near the close of this book, the questions that probably continue to burn in your mind concern prevention. We have touched on many aspects of prevention. But it is such an important topic, both to you and to me, that a chapter devoted to the many ways you can protect yourself and your loved ones against HPV is in order.

Perhaps the following story will bring home my reasons for feeling so passionate about prevention:

Barbara was a healthy married woman in her late twenties. A member of the military, she was stationed in Germany for three years. She dutifully went for checkups annually and had Pap testing. All her Pap smears were normal.

During the last year in Germany, her Pap smear results were very disturbing. The military physician found a high-grade lesion. Since her tour of duty was about to end, and she was only days away from her return to the United States, the doctors in Germany told her to make an appointment as soon as possible with her own physician at home and to show him her test results.

Barbara complied. But instead of performing a colposcopy and biopsy, her doctor performed another Pap smear, the results of which were normal. He sent her home with a clean bill of health, telling her that clearly the doctors overseas were incompetent.

Relieved and overjoyed, Barbara began planning for the future. She became pregnant and delivered a healthy baby. All seemed to be going well until after delivery, when her bleeding did not stop. On examination, her doctor discovered a large cervical lesion. Biopsy revealed that she had rapidly progressing invasive squamous cancer. Her medical team was unable to stop the progression of the disease, and Barbara died shortly before her baby's first birthday.

Why have I chosen this story to illustrate this point? Clearly, there are aspects of gross medical mismanagement of this patient's care. And certainly, this case is a horrible tragedy resulting in the death of a young woman before she even knew her child well. But to me, the added dimension of this tragedy was that a more educated patient could have taken different steps and interrupted the disease progression at many points along the way. Compare her story to those in Chapters 5 and 6, where informed patients insisted on proper follow-up of disturbing Pap smear results. If at each juncture this patient had been knowledgeable about the meaning of her diagnosis, she might have banged on her physician's desk and demanded proper treatment. The progression of Barbara's illness could have been arrested anywhere along the way with some proactive management.

So the first and most important aspect of prevention is education. You have already taken that step by reading this book. Let's continue then by looking at ways you can reduce the risk of contracting HPV. If you already have been infected, the suggestions in this chapter might help prevent the virus from doing further damage. Remember that only a small percentage of those infected with HPV will go on to develop genital warts, cervical disease, or cervical cancer. It may even be possible to vanquish the virus from the body altogether! Until recently, we assumed that complete eradication of HPV was unlikely. However, we have not been absolutely certain of this because our ability to test for the virus has not been around for that long. Now that we have a reliable test for the virus, we has discovered that increasing numbers of women have "cleared" the virus from their bodies—that is, brought the levels of the virus down so low that it is undetectable in a laboratory test.

Your ability to reduce the risk of infection, prevent the virus from progressing and becoming symptomatic, and get rid of it altogether will depend on the strength of your immune system—which, in turn, is closely related to your lifestyle choices. This chapter will review what we know about these choices. The suggestions below should therefore provide hope for you and for other women with whom you are in contact.

Establish Good Nutrition Habits

As you learned in Chapter 10, good nutrition is a cornerstone of a preventive program. It builds the immune system so that if you are infected with HPV, you do not necessarily go on to develop genital warts or cervical disease. If you already have these conditions, adequate nutrition may tip the balance between the worsening of your symptoms and the arresting or even reversing of your disease progression.

Years ago, children were taught about the "four basic food groups" in school. Today we speak of a "food pyramid." Adapting the concept of the food pyramid, vegetables and fruits should form the base of the pyramid, or the staple of your diet. Vegetables are rich in dietary antioxidants such as beta-carotene and vitamins A, C, and E. Numerous studies have shown that a diet high in fresh fruits and the full range of vegetables—especially leafy green and cruciferous vegetables—lowers the risk of all kinds of cancer, not to mention cardiovascular disease and other ailments. And remember that wonderful new compound—I3C—which is derived from cruciferous vegetables. Increased risk of cervical disease has specifically been associated with deficiencies in vitamins A, B, and C, and folic acid.

A healthy diet should also include plenty of complex carbohydrates, such as whole-grain products and lots of protein. Egg whites, low-fat dairy products, and lean meat and poultry are excellent sources of protein. Even better are fish products, which contain beneficial essential fatty acids (EFAs), and soy protein and chickpeas, which contain plant-based estrogens that help balance estrogen levels in the body. Nuts and seeds also contain protein.

Refined flour products, such as white bread and pasta; fatty foods, such as ice cream and fried foods; fatty meats; and refined sugar products, such as candy and cake, should be significantly limited. They cause undesirable weight gain, which is not only a cosmetic problem, but also a health problem. Fat cells are like storage facilities for estrogen. Remember that estrogen dominance has been implicated in the development of cervical disease. Moreover, these foods overtax the body's digestive and metabolic systems. High-fat diets have been associated with increased risk of many types of cancer.

Vitamin and mineral supplementation can help ensure that you're getting enough of these vital micronutrients on a daily basis. Because of today's farming techniques, some of our vegetables and fruits are not as packed with nutrients as they used to be—assuming we're eating enough of them to provide us with necessary nutrients, which most of us aren't. Vitamin and mineral supplementation is an excellent way to play it safe.

QUIT SMOKING

Anti-smoking campaigns have been around for a long time and the association between smoking and lung cancer is well established, both in the professional community and in the awareness of the lay public. Many people don't know that smoking can increase the risk of contracting other types of cancer as well—including cervical cancer. Smoking is not just associated with increased risk of cervical cancer but also with poorer success at clearing HPV from the system, arresting the progression of cervical dysplasia, and ensuring that genital warts don't recur once they have been treated. A June 2001 study in the *Journal of the American Medical Association* examined numerous potential risk factors related to the development and persistence of LGSIL. Out of all of them, which do you think was the worst? That's right. Smoking. In fact, the more research that's done, the more aware we become that smoking has no "up" side, and more "down" sides than we ever imagined.

So if you're a smoker, it's time to quit. There are many excellent programs available both online and in person to assist you. Contact the American Lung Association or the American Cancer Society for further information.

OVERCOME SUBSTANCE ABUSE

Like smoking, alcohol and drug abuse have been implicated as a cause of a variety of conditions. Alcoholism causes cirrhosis of the liver. Even drinkers whose livers do not degenerate to that point can damage their livers in less dramatic, subtler ways. As mentioned in Chapter 10, the liver is an important organ in the efficient processing of female hormones and in maintaining good hormonal health. Additionally, sexual risk-taking behaviors are often associated with altered states of consciousness. People who are high on drugs often do not take adequate sexual precautions. Drug abuse is associated with a larger number of sexual partners, probably because people who are drunk or high do not carefully think through their decisions and are more likely to rush into sexual liaisons. Remember that multiple partners is one of the most significant risk factors for contracting HPV and also for having that virus progress to cervical dysplasia.

Being free of addiction to alcohol and drugs can only enhance your health and overall well-being in every area of your life. You can get help by contacting a counselor or mental health center with a specialty in substance abuse issues by contacting the National Drug Council or by contacting Alcoholics Anonymous or Narcotics Anonymous.

TAKE SEXUAL PRECAUTIONS

While taking sexual precautions is certainly the most obvious way to prevent infection by a sexually transmitted disease such as HIV, the nature of the precautions that we should take are less clear with the HPV virus. As we have discussed, better known methods such as condom usage are not effective in preventing HPV. Certainly, the safe sex practices designed to protect against the transmission of the HIV virus are a starting point. Here are a few additional suggestions.

LIMIT YOUR SEX PARTNERS

As I've said before, in this case, sexual promiscuity isn't a moral issue, it's a medical issue. The more partners you have, the more vulnerable you become to infection by HPV and to its progression into genital warts, cervical dysplasia, or even cervical cancer. So many people are viral carriers (often without symptoms) that you may be infected with multiple strains. It's as if you were stung by a swarm of bees, each with a slightly different variety of venom. Some strains might be relatively innocuous, but some may be high risk. It stands to reason that every time you are intimate with someone who has HPV, you reintroduce it into your body, or you import new strains. The greater the viral load, the harder your immune system has to work, and the more symptoms you might develop.

AVOID SEXUAL CONTACT WITH PEOPLE WHO
HAVE HAD MULTIPLE SEX PARTNERS

For the same reason that multiple sex partners are a risk factor for you, they are also a risk factor for your partner. While inquiry into someone's sexual past does not always produce an honest answer, it's at least worth a try to get some profile of the individual with whom you are considering sharing your body. When you think a new relationship might become sexual, you should discuss with each other your sexual history before you do anything more than kiss.

MAKE SURE YOUR SEX PARTNER IS TREATED
IF YOU HAVE BEEN DIAGNOSED

If you have genital warts or a cervical condition associated with HPV, your sex partner will almost certainly have been exposed to the virus, and there is a strong chance that he may develop the symptoms of infection. For his sake and for yours, make sure he is examined and treated if necessary. Remember that men are far more frequently asymptomatic carriers than are women. Inspecting his genital area and finding it free of lesions does not prove that he is free of the virus.

DO NOT ASSUME THAT YOU ARE IMMUNE
TO INFECTION IF YOU ARE A LESBIAN

As we have seen, HPV is communicated through skin-to-skin contact—which is what sex, including lesbian sex, is all about.

AVOID ORAL SEX WITH AN INFECTED PARTNER

You are likely to be wondering about HPV and oral sex. As we have discussed in earlier chapters, several HPV strains can infect the mouth and the respiratory tract, with diseases such as recurrent respiratory papillomatosis (RRP) resulting. Once thought to be a disease of children only, RRP is now being seen with increasing frequency in adults in their twenties and thirties. The suspected mechanism is oral sex. In addition, recent studies have also shown that as much as 30 percent of head and neck cancers may be HPV-related. Given this new, somewhat alarming data, it seems wise to avoid oral sex with partners known to be infected with HPV.

I realize that some of these recommendations are somewhat vague and may also be alarming, not to mention inconvenient and disruptive to sexual practices and patterns you have already established. Perhaps this is one reason for the persistent silence on the part of public medical educators regarding this virus. First of all, we don't yet have complete concrete information to offer. How many sex partners are "too many"? Is oral sex really unsafe? As difficult as the public campaign for safe sex to prevent the spread of HIV has been, this is even more daunting because there are few clear guidelines to offer. Remember that even fondling, petting, and other forms of intimate sexual contact without intercourse may be high-risk behavior. All I can say is that scientists are intensively investigating these issues. I am hopeful that more extensive and specific guidelines will be available in the future. Until then, my clinical experience has led me to offer the foregoing and following suggestions.

PRACTICE SENSIBLE HYGIENE

There is now some evidence that HPV can be transmitted through *fomites*—inanimate objects that have touched the virus. These include sex toys, tanning beds, and even toilet seats. The question hinges on the extent to which the virus can survive outside of its human host. Many viruses, such as HIV, cannot survive under these conditions. Although some people have contracted HPV from sex toys and tanning beds, we still do not know how extensive this method of transmission is, particularly by toilet seats. We do know that HPV is a remarkable and frighteningly hardy organism. In the past, some physicians who performed laser vaporization on genital warts developed respiratory papillomatosis some years after the procedure. It turned out that the vaporized virus continued to live in the air, and when these physicians inhaled, their respiratory tract became infected. Now doctors wear special protective masks.

So be cautious and be sensible. Cover toilet seats in public places. Don't share sex paraphernalia. Wash new underwear and bathing suits, which may have been tried on by someone infected by the virus. Ask for a protective covering on tanning tables, sauna benches, and similar places. If you know you have genital warts and have touched your genitals, wash your hands so you don't communicate the virus to others—including your children. Keep generally clean and be careful about sharing soap with someone who might be infected.

These measures may seem excessive. It may be that in a few years, as research into this virus progresses, we will have enough information to breathe a sigh of relief and say that you can't be infected by fomites. Right now, I can only advise erring on the side of caution in this area as well as in other areas.

ENGAGE IN PHYSICAL EXERCISE

Numerous studies have shown that physical exercise is an important component of good health. The sedentary lifestyle many Americans lead today is known to contribute to numerous ailments, including cardiovascular disease and all types of cancer. Exercise tones the system, builds muscle, increases efficient blood flow, and thereby strengthens immunity. It also helps people to feel better. Studies have shown that exercise has mildly antidepressant qualities and that it increases the *endorphins* or feel-good chemicals in the brain. If you are working to build your health, you will want to include a basic exercise program in your lifestyle. And if you have been diagnosed with an illness, exercise will help you to feel better both physically and emotionally.

HAVE AN ANNUAL PAP TEST

By now you know that the single most effective way of preventing cervical cancer is by having an annual Pap test. The neglect of this important screening test leads to the progression of an illness that could have been detected early, or prevented in the first place. There is no reason for this to happen. All insurers cover the costs of a conventional Pap smear and an increasing number of insurance companies are covering the cost of monolayer Pap tests and HPV testing. The test is quick, simple, painless, and noninvasive. It provides crucial information about the state of your cervix. If you are stressed for time or money and are cutting corners, don't make the annual Pap smear a "cut" corner!

In general, having an annual gynecological examination can protect you not only from cervical cancer but also from other conditions, particularly HPV-related conditions. If you have an early case of genital warts, a gynecologist can spot and treat them before they spread too far or become too large. Checkups are a very helpful way to make sure that small problems are nipped in the bud before they become big problems.

Delaying Sexual Activity— Educating Youngsters

It has been demonstrated in study after study that sex at an early age creates greater susceptibility to cervical dysplasia. Teenagers are notoriously difficult to work with. The "terrible teens" can be as trying as the "terrible twos." This is the age when youngsters are rebelling, trying to carve out an independent identity, and the last thing they want to hear about is another limitation on their newfound sexual experimentation. It's been hard enough to get them to use condoms!

If you are a parent or teacher, you might find that educating teens about genital warts could be more helpful than telling them about cervical cancer. They'll see cervical cancer as some ailment they don't really have to worry about now, as irrelevant to them as grandma's arthritis. But teens are very appearance-conscious and are sensitive to things that are "gross." They will see genital warts as "gross" and unattractive. Their anxiety about their appearance can be a more powerful deterrent than all the cancer-focused campaigns in the world. Consider how marginally effective the anti-smoking campaigns have been with this age group. But if teens believed that smoking caused huge, cauliflowerlike lesions on the face necessitating removal with a laser or painful medication, you can be sure Joe Camel would pose little threat.

The longer sexual activity is delayed the greater a young women's chances of having a healthy cervix. Similarly, every month of abstinence for a young male is a month in which he is not contracting or spreading the disease. So it's really a matter of buying time. Consider each month of deferred sexual activity to be an accomplishment.

TALK TO YOUR PARTNER

If you are in a relationship, your partner's support and involvement with this program to change your lifestyle will be very important. Often, it can spell the difference between success and failure to implement important changes. It is difficult to cook and eat differently if your partner does not understand what you are doing or why. If your body image has changed as a result of your diagnosis—many women feel less attractive—then share this with your partner. He can reassure you that you are still loved and that the presence of a virus does not make you less desirable. However, if this does become an obstacle in your relationship, consider entering conjugal counseling, as discussed before. The more open you are in communicating your fears, concerns, needs, and wants, the closer you can become.

Other issues to raise with your partner concern his own need for treatment or at least evaluation, since he has been exposed to you and may well be infected. A positive way to envision this time is as a way to grow closer. If you are sharing this disease, you are also sharing this battle with the disease and the process could serve to unite you even more.

GET PSYCHOLOGICAL COUNSELING IF NECESSARY

Lifestyle changes are difficult to initiate and even more difficult to maintain. Old habits die hard, and altering your lifestyle can feel like a daunting task. My advice is to initiate changes gradually, one step at a time, so you don't get overwhelmed. Some sessions with an experienced counselor—psychologist or social worker—might help you to identify issues that are tripping you up and help you put strategies in place to maximize your chances of success.

Counseling is particularly important if you've received a troubling diagnosis or even a troubling test result on a Pap smear. One of the most neglected wounds of HPV-related infection are the psychological wounds. Receiving any difficult diagnosis is hard, but a diagnosis of a sexually transmitted disease is particularly difficult. Numerous studies have shown that the diagnosis of an STD may cause a lot of stress. In my opinion, many of the current "approved" management strategies for treatment rely on long periods of repeated Pap smears, which often prolong the uncertainty and agony. It is emotionally difficult to deal with a diagnosis such as HPV, a potential problem such as ASCUS, an unpleasant condition such as genital warts, or a life-threatening condition such as cervical cancer. Psychological issues you might face include:

- Dealing with altered body image—seeing yourself as damaged or unattractive;
- Dealing with sexual challenges and taking better care of yourself;
- Developing motivation and commitment to make necessary dietary and lifestyle changes and putting good intentions into action;
- Giving up addictions, such as cigarette smoking, alcohol, and drugs;
- Presenting these issues to your partner.

If you are facing cancer, a support group can be an invaluable environment to help you confront the myriad psychological issues that are likely to arise.

"AN OUNCE OF PREVENTION IS WORTH A POUND OF CURE"

The best treatment for HPV-related conditions is a good preventive program that helps you avoid contracting these conditions to begin with. The more people who practice prevention and educate others, the more we will begin to reverse the alarming rise of HPV in this country and, indeed, worldwide. But if you have been diagnosed with an HPV-associated condition, don't despair. You can still prevent it from worsening and you can prevent others from catching it.

12

Conclusions and Future Directions

I have described HPV as the virus no one ever told you about. By now you have been told plenty about it! You know what it is, how it invades the body, and what damage it can do. This knowledge can make an enormous difference in your life. You can use it to protect yourself against the virus as much as possible, to treat the virus if you already have it, and to protect yourself from its harmful and deadly effects.

As much as you know, and as much as is known by physicians and scientists devoted to researching this virus, it doesn't compare to what is unknown. In fact, it is the magnitude of what we do not know that has made the writing of this book so difficult. Telling the public what they need to know about this virus in a manner that is accessible, comprehensible, and informative and that promotes action, protection, and prevention (rather than mass panic) has felt like a Herculean task. This would have been the case even if HPV were just *one* virus. But because it's actually a *family* of viruses with a variety of effects at a variety of bodily sites, and its effects are so profoundly connected with so many other risk factors, writing this book became even more daunting. Perhaps this is one of the reasons why far more distinguished scientists than I, who have devoted their entire lives to studying this virus, have not written a book about it.

I hope that I've succeeded in accomplishing the goal of *Women at Risk,* which is not only to help you, the individual reader, but also to make the public aware of the existence of HPV and its alarming rampage through the population. If trends continue, today's 60 to 80 percent infected may become tomorrow's 80 to 100 percent. This can lead to an increase not only in cervical disease and genital warts but also in respiratory papillomatosis among young children who have been exposed to the virus.

All this sounds very grim. But the good news it that scientists are increasing their efforts to understand this virus and develop ways to both treat and prevent it. Researchers are discovering new strains of the virus. Some studies now suggest the possibility that certain strains are normal, harmless inhabitants of the genital tract and may, in fact, be beneficial by stimulating the immune system to fight the more dangerous strains. If these beneficial types could be sorted out and distinguished from the destructive types, we could understand better how to build the immune system and assist it in combating the invasion of the unhealthy types.

In my opinion, our greatest hope lies in the development of an effective vaccine, and this has not gone unnoticed by drug companies. Many of them are devoting huge resources to developing such vaccines. In February 2001, a study conducted at the National Institutes of Health was released. It confirmed the effectiveness of a vaccine against HPV type 16. Even though it can only provide immunity against one strain of the virus (although a particularly virulent strain, as you will recall), it can assist in combating other viral strains by reducing the total viral load. It seems likely that this vaccination will receive FDA approval and become part of routine health care some time in the near future.

So the future isn't as grim as would appear. Each day new scientific advances give hope for a way to prevent the spread of HPV and to treat those who have already been infected. "The future" is a vague term and lies someplace on the distant horizon. It's very easy to sit back and say that "they" are researching HPV and when "they" find a vaccine or cure, the disease incidence will decrease. Relying on others, even distinguished scientists, isn't enough. Each one of you reading this book is now armed with the most effective tool that we now have in the war against HPV—education. And now you can become an educator and thereby participate in this war. It is important for each of you to play a role in educating others about this disease. If you are in the medical or allied health professions, if you are in the military, or if you are a teacher, you're in a position to directly affect the lives of others by disseminating information and educating those with whom you work. And even if you're not in one of these fields, you can still have an impact on others. If you tell your friends and they, in turn, inform their friends, the information will spread by word of mouth. (Think of the movie *Pay It Forward,* in which dramatic societal change was brought about by a single boy.)

My contribution to the war on HPV is this book. By purchasing it, you have already taken a step in aiding this cause. A major portion of the proceeds from the sale of the book will be used to start a foundation devoted to HPV diagnosis, research, and awareness. The foundation will be devoted to helping cover the cost of newer diagnostic methods for women who cannot afford them; sponsoring scientific research projects aimed at finding cures from HPV-related diseases; and promoting awareness campaigns at the community and national level. It is my dream that one day a national effort of the magnitude of the

"Race for the Cure" campaign against breast cancer by the Komen foundation will be launched against the global HPV epidemic. I thank you for your contribution to making this dream a reality.

As much as we still don't know, we do know that HPV is a sexually transmitted disease that is the cause of a number of cancerous conditions and life-threatening noncancerous conditions. That knowledge empowers us to prevent most of these diseases and, indeed, to hold the hope that all of these diseases can be completely eradicated in the future. If you will join me in getting that message through to the American public, you will be ensuring a safer, healthier society not only for you, but for your children and grandchildren as well.

References

Ambros, R. A., and Kurman, R. J. Current concepts in the relationship of human papillomavirus infection to the pathogenesis and classification of precancerous squamous lesions of the uterine cervix. *Semin. Diagn. Pathol.* 1990, 7:158–172.

Anderson, M. C. Glandular lesions of the cervix. In: Jones, H. W., ed., *Cervical Intraepithelial Neoplasia.* London: Billierre Tindall, 1995, 9:105–119.

Anderson, M. C. Premalignant and malignant squamous lesions of the cervix. In: Fox, H., and Wells, M., eds. *Haines and Taylor's Obstetrical and Gynaecological Pathology,* 4th ed. New York: Churchill Livingstone, 1995, 292–297.

Antoni, M., Goodkin, K., Helder, L. Psychosocial stressors, coping, and cervical neoplasia in 3 sample studies from 1981–1990. In *12th Annual Scientific Sessions of the Society of Behavioral Medicine.* Rockville, Md.: Society of Behavioral Medicine, 991:281.

Arany, I., and Tyring, S. K. Activation of local cell-mediated immunity in interferon-responsive patients with human papillomavirus-associated lesions. *J. Interferon Cytokine Res.* 1996, 16:453–460.

Austin, R. M. Results of blinded rescreening of Papanicolaou smears versus biased retrospective review. *Arch. Pathol. Lab Med.* 1997, 121:311–314.

Barton, S. E., Maddox, P. H., Jenkins, D., Edwards, R., Cuzick, J., and Singer, A. Effect of cigarette smoking on cervical epithelial immunity: A mechanism for neoplastic change? *Lancet* 1988, 2:652–654.

Basu, J., et al. Smoking and the antioxidant ascorbic acid: plasma, leukocyte and cervicovaginal cell concentrations in normal healthy women. *Am. J. Obstet Gynecol* 1990, Dec., 163 (6 Pt1):1948–1952.

Basu, J., Paln, P., Vermund, S., et al. Plasma ascorbic acid and beta carotene levels in women evaluated for HPV infection, smoking and cervix dysplasia. *Canc Detect Prev* 1991, 15:165–70.

Bauer, H. M., Hildersheim, A., Schiffman, M. H., et al. Determinants of genital human papillomavirus infection in low-risk women in Portland, Oregon. *Sex. Transm. Dis.* 1993, 20:274–277.

Bauer, H. M., Ting, Y., Greer, C. E., et al. Genital human papillomavirus infection in female university students as determined by a PCR-based method. *JAMA* 1991, 265:472–477.

Bauman, N. M., and Smith, R. J. Recurrent respiratory papillomatosis. *Pediatric Clinics of North America* 1996, 43(6):1385–1401.

Bibbo, M., et al. Performance of the AutoPap primary screening system at Jefferson University. *Acta Cytol.* 1999, 43:27–29.

Birley, H. D. Human papillomaviruses, cervical cancer and the developing world. *Anls. Tropical. Med. Parasitol* 1995, 89:453–463.

Bishop, J. W., Kaufman, R. H., and Taylor, D. A. Multicenter comparison of manual and automated screening of AutoCyte gynecologic preparations. *Acta Cytol.* 1999, 43:34–38.

Bishop, J. W., Bigner, S. H., Colgan, T. J., Husain, M., et al. Multicenter masked evaluation of AutoCyte PREP thin layers with matched conventional smears. *Acta Cytol.* 1998, 42:189–197.

Bogdanich, W. Lax laboratories: The Pap test misses much cervical cancer through lab's errors. *The Wall Street Journal,* 1987.

Bogdanich, W. Physician's carelessness with Pap test is cited in procedure's high failure rate. *The Wall Street Journal,* 1987.

Boronow, R. C. Death of the Papanicolaou smear? A tale of three reasons. *Am. J. Obstet Gynecol.* 1998, 179:391–396.

Boronow, R. C., et al. When your patient asks: "Doctor, I read there have been serious Pap smear errors. Shouldn't I get one of those new computer Pap smears?" *J. Miss. State Med. Assoc.* 1998, 34:136–141.

Bosch, F. X., Manos, M. M., Munoz, N., et al., and the International Biological Study on Cervical Cancer (IBSCC) Study Group. Prevalence of human papillomavirus in cervical cancer: A worldwide perspective. *J. Nat. Cancer. Inst.* 1995, 87:796–802.

Brinton, L. Oral contraceptives and cervical neoplasia. *Contr* 1991, 43:581.

Brown, A. D., and Garber, A. Cost-effectiveness of 3 methods to enhance the sensitivity of Papanicolaou testing. *JAMA* 1999, 281:347–353.

Burk, R. D. Pernicious papillomavirus infection. *N. Eng. J. Med.* 1999, 341: 1687–1688.

Butterworth, C. E. Effect of folate on cervical cancer. *Beyond Deficiencies* 1992, 293–299.

Butterworth, C. E., Hatch, K. D., Macaluso, M., et al. Folate deficiency and cervical dysplasia. *JAMA* 1992, 267:528–533.

Campion, M. J., Brown, J. R., McCance, D. L., et al. Psychosexual trauma of an abnormal Pap smear. *Br. J. Obstet. Gynecol.* 1988, 95:175–181.

Campion, M. J., Ferris, D. G., Reid, R. R., et al. *Modern Colposcopy.* Hagerstown, MD: American Society for Colposcopy and Cervical Pathology, 1995.

Chamberlain, J. Reasons that some screening programs fail to control cervical cancer. In: Hakama, M., Miller, A. B., and Day, N. E., eds., *Screening for Cancer of the Uterine Cervix* (IARC Scientific Publications No. 76). Lyon: IARC Scientific Publications, 1992, 161–168.

Chichareon, S., Herrero, R., Munoz, N., et al. Risk factors for cervical cancer in Thailand: A case control study. *J. Natl. Cancer Inst.* 1998, 90:50–57.

Clarke, E. A., Hatcher, J., McKeown-Eyssen, G. E., and Lickrish, G. M. Cervical dysplasia association with sexual behavior, smoking, and oral contraceptive use? *Am. J. Obstet. Gynecol.* 1985, 151:612–616.

Clavel, C., Masure, M., Bory, J.-P., Putaud, I., Mangeonjean, C., et al. Hybrid Capture II-based human papillomavirus detection, a sensitive test to detect in routine high-grade cervical lesions: A preliminary study on 1518 women. *B. J. Cancer* 1999, 80:1306–1311.

Clavel, C., Masure, M., Putaud, I., et al. Hybrid Capture® II, a new sensitive test for human papillomavirus detection: Comparison with hybrid capture I and PCR results in cervical lesions. *J. Clin. Pathol.* 1998, 51:737–740.

Coker, A., McCann, M., Hulka, B., et al. Oral contraceptive use and cervical intraepithelial neoplasia. *J Clin Epid* 1992, 45(10) 1111.

Corkill, M., Knapp, D., and Hutchinson, M. L. Improved accuracy for cervical cytology with the ThinPrep method and the endocervical brush-spatula collection procedure. *J. Lower Genital Tract Dis.* 1998, 2:12–16.

Cox, J. T. AGUS Pap smears: A follow-up strategy. *OBG Management* 1998, 7:74–87.

Cox, J. T. ASCCP practice guideline: Management of glandular abnormalities in the cervical smear. *J. Lower Gen. Tract Dis.* 1997, 1:41–45.

Cox, J. T. Clinical utility of HPV testing. In: Lorincz, A. T., ed. *Obstetrics and Gynecology Clinics of North America.* Philadelphia: W. B. Saunders, 1996, 23(4): 811–852.

Cox, J. T. The epidemiology of CIN—What is the role of HPV? In: *Ballieres Clinical Obstetrics and Gynecology.* London: Balliere Tindall, 1995, 9:1–37.

Cox, J. T. Evaluating the role of HPV testing for women with equivocal Papanicolaou test findings. *JAMA* 1999, 281:1645–1647.

Cox, J. T., Lonky, N., Tosh, R., and Massad, S. ASCCP practice guideline: Management of low-grade squamous intraepithelial lesion (LSIL). *J. Lower Gen. Tract Dis.* 2000, 4:83–92.

Cox, J. T., Lorincz, A. T., Schiffman, M. H., et al. HPV testing by hybrid capture appears to be useful in triaging women with a cytologic diagnosis of ASCUS. *Am. J. Obstet. Gynecol.* 1995, 172:946–954.

Cox, J. T., Schiffman, M. H., Winzelberg, A. J., and Patterson, J. M. An evaluation of human papillomavirus testing as part of referral to colposcopy clinics. *Obstet. Gynecol.* 1992, 80:389–395.

Cox, J. T., Wilkinson, E., Lonky, N., Waxman, A., Tosh, R., and Tedeschi, C. ASCCP practice guideline: Management guidelines for follow-up of atypical squamous cells of undetermined significance (ASCUS). *J. Lower Gen. Tract Dis.* 2000, 4:99–113.

Cuzick, J., Szarewski, A., Terry, G., et al. Human papillomavirus testing in primary cervical cancer screening. *Lancet* 1995, 345:1533–1536.

Daling, J. R., Madeleine, M. M., McKnight, B., et al. The relationship of human papillomavirus-related cervical tumors to cigarette smoking, oral contraceptive use, and prior herpes simplex virus type 2 infection. *Cancer Epidemiol. Biomarkers Prev.* 1996, 5:541–548.

Demay, R. M. Common problems in Papanicolaou smear interpretation. *Arch. Pathol. Lab Med.* 1997, 121:229–238.

Derkay, C. S. Task force on recurrent respiratory papillomatosis. *Arch. Otolaryng. Head Neck Surg.* 1995, 121:1386–1391.

Deskin, R. W. Laser laryngoscopy for papilloma removal. In: Bailey, B. J., et al., *Atlas of Head and Neck Surgery—Otolaryngology.* Lippincott-Raven, 1998.

De Vet, H. C., Knipschild, P. G., and Sturmans, F. The role of sexual factors in the aetiology of cervical dysplasia. *Int. J. Epidemiol.* 1993, 22:798–803.

Diaz-Rosario, L. A., and Kabawat, S. E. Performance of a fluid-based, thin-layer Papanicolaou smear method in the clinical setting of an independent laboratory and an outpatient screening population in New England. *Arch. Pathol. Lab. Med.* 1999, 123:817–821.

Duska, L. R., Flynn, C. F., Chen, A., et al. Clinical evaluation of atypical glandular cells of undetermined significance on cervical cytology. *Obstet. Gynecol.* 1998, 91:278–282.

Eddy, G. L., Strumpf, K. B., Wojtowycz, M. A., et al. Biopsy findings in 531 patients with atypical glandular cells of undetermined significance (AGCUS) as defined by the Bethesda System (TBS). *Am. J. Obstet. Gynecol.* 1997, 177:1188–1195.

Fahey, M. T., Irwig, L., and Macaskill, P. Meta-analysis of Pap test accuracy. *Am. J. Epidemiol.* 1995, 141:680–689.

Ferenczy, A., and Jenson, A. B. Tissue effects and host response: The key to the rational triage of cervical neoplasia. *Obstet. Gynecol. Clin. North Am.* 1996, 23:759–782.

Gabbott, M., Cossart, Y. E., Kan, A., Konopka, M., Chan, R., and Rose, B. R. Human papillomavirus and host variables as predictors of clinical course in patients with juvenile-onset recurrent respiratory papillomatosis. *J. Clin. Microbiol.* 1997, 35:3098–3103.

Gaylis, B., and Hayden, R. E. Recurrent respiratory papillomatosis: Progression to invasion and malignancy. *Am. J. Otolaryng.* 1991, 12(2):104–112.

Harahap, R. E. Influence of sexual activity on development of cervical intraepithelial neoplasia (CIN). *Cancer Detect. Prev.* 1986, 9:237–241.

Harro, C. D., Pang, Y. Y., Roden, R. B., Hildesheim, A., Wang, Z., et al. Safety and immunogenicity trial in adult volunteers of a human papillomavirus 16 L1 virus-like particle vaccine. *J. Natl. Cancer Inst.* 2001, 93:284–292.

Healy, G. B., Gelber, R. D., Trowbridge, A. L., et al. Treatment of recurrent respiratory papillomatosis with human leukocyte interferon. *N. Eng. J. Med.* 1988, 319:401–407.

Hellberg, D., Nilsson, S., and Valentin, J. Positive cervical smear with subsequent normal colposcopy and histology—frequency of CIN in a long-term follow-up. *Gynecol. Oncol.* 1994, 53:148–151.

Ho, G. Y. F., Bierman, R., Beardsley, L., Chang, C. J., and Burk, R. D. Natural history of cervicovaginal papillomavirus infection in young women. *N. Engl. J. Med.* 1998, 338:4233–428.

Ho, G. Y. F., Burk, R. D., Klein, S., et al. Persistent genital human papillomavirus infection as a risk factor for persistent cervical dysplasia. *J. Natl. Cancer Inst.* 1995, 87:1365–1371.

Hutchinson, M. L., Isenstein, L. M., Goodman, A., Hurley, A. A., et al. Homogeneous sampling accounts for the increased diagnostic accuracy using the ThinPrep processor. *Am. J. Clin. Pathol.* 1994, 101:215–219.

Hutchinson, M., Zahniser, D., Sherman, M. E., Herrero, R., et al. Utility of liquid-based cytology for cervical cancer screening: Results of a population-based study conducted in a high cervical cancer incidence region of Costa Rica. *Cancer Cytopath.* 1999.

Kadish, A. S., Ho, G. Y., Burk, R. D., et al. Lymphoproliferative responses to human papillomavirus (HPV) type 16 proteins E6 and E7: Outcome of HPV infection and associated neoplasia. *J. Natl. Cancer Inst.* 1997, 89:1285–1293.

Kainz, C., Tempfer, C., Gitsch, G., et al. Influence of age and human papillomavirus infection on reliability of cervical cytology. *Arch. Gynecol. Obstet.* 1995, 256:23–28.

Kashima, H. K., Mounts, P., and Shah, K. Recurrent respiratory papillomatosis. *Obs. Gyn. Clin. of N. Am.* 1996, 23(3):699–706.

Kataja, V., Syrjonen, S., Mantyiarvi, R., Yliskoski, M., Saarikoski, S., and Syrjonen, K. Prognostic factors in cervical human papillomavirus infections. *Sex. Transm. Dis.* 1992, 19:154–160.

Kato, I., Santamaria, M., De Ruiz, P. A., et al. Interobserver variation in cytological and histological diagnoses of cervical neoplasia and its epidemiologic implication. *J. Clin. Epidemiol.* 1995, 48:1167–1174.

Kennedy, A. W., Salmieri, S. S., Wirth, S. L., et al. Results of the clinical evaluation of atypical glandular cells of undetermined significance (AGCUS) detected on cervical cytology screening. *Gynecol. Oncol.* 1996, 63:14–18.

Kinny, W. K., Manos, M. M., Hurley, L. B., and Ransley, J. E. Where's the high-grade cervical neoplasia? The importance of the minimally abnormal Papanicolaou diagnosis. *Obstet. Gynecol.* 1998, 91:973–976.

Kiser, S. K., van den Brule, A. J. C., Bock, J. E., et al. Human papillomavirus: The most significant risk determinant of cervical intraepithelial neoplasia. *Int. J. Cancer* 1996, 65:601–606.

Kosko, J. R., and Derkay, C. S. Role of cesarean section in prevention of recurrent respiratory papillomatosis—is there one? *Int. J. Ped. Otorhinolaryng.* 1996, 35(1):31–38.

Kost, L. G. The Papanicolaou test for cervical cancer detection: A triumph and a tragedy. *JAMA* 1989, 261:737–743.

Koutsky, L. A., for the ALTS Group. HPV triage as a management strategy for women with low-grade squamous intraepithelial lesions. *J. Natl. Cancer Inst.* 2000.

Koutsky, L. A., Holmes, K. K., Critchlow, C. W., et al. A cohort study of the risks of cervical intraepithelial neoplasia grade 2 or 3 in relation to papillomavirus infection. *N. Engl. J. Med.* 1992, 327:1272–1278.

Kurman, R. J., Henson, D., Herbst, A., Noller, K., and Schiffman, M. H.. Interim guidelines for management of abnormal cervical cytology. *JAMA* 1994, 271:1866–1869.

Kurman, R. J., and Solomon, D. *The Bethesda System for Reporting Cervical/Vaginal Cytologic Diagnoses. Definitions, Criteria, and Explanatory Notes for Terminology and Specimen Adequacy.* New York: Springer Verlag, 1993.

Laimins, L. A. Review. The biology of human papillomaviruses: From warts to cancer. *Infect. Agents. Dis.* 1994, 2:74–86.

La Vecchia, C., Franceschi, S., Decarli, A., et al. Sexual factors, venereal diseases, and risk of intraepithelial and invasive cervical neoplasia. *Cancer* 1986, 58:935–941.

Lee, K., Ashfaq, R., Birdsong, G. G., Corkill, M. E., McIntosh, K. M., and Inhorn, S. L. Comparison of conventional Papanicolaou smears and a fluid-based, thin-layer system for cervical cancer screening. *Obstet. Gynecol.* 1997, 90:278–284.

Lee, K. R., Minter, L. J., and Crum, C. P. Koilocytotic atypia in Papanicolaou smears: Reproducibility and biopsy correlation. *Cancer Cytopathol.* 1997, 81:10–15.

Liaw, K. L., Glass, A. G., Manos, M. M., et al. Detection of human papillomavirus DNA in cytologically normal women and subsequent cervical squamous intraepithelial lesions. *J. Natl. Cancer Inst.* 1999, 91:954–960.

Lorincz, A. Molecular methods for the detection of human papillomavirus infection. In: Lorincz, A., and Reid, R., eds., *Human Papillomavirus I.* Philadelphia: W. B. Saunders, 1996.

Manos, M. M., Kinney, W. K., Hurley, L. B., et al. Identifying women with cervical neoplasia: Using human papillomavirus testing for equivocal Papanicolaou results. *JAMA* 1999, 281:1605–1610.

Mayeaux, E. J., Harper, M. B., Abreo, F., et al. A comparison of the reliability of repeat cervical smears and colposcopy in patients with abnormal cervical cytology. *J. Fam. Prac.* 1995, 40:57–62.

Meijer, C. J., Helmerhorst, T. J., Rozendaal, L., van der Linden, J. C., Voorhorst, F. J., and Walboomers, J. M. Human papillomavirus typing or testing in gynacopathology: Has the time come? *Histopathology* 1998, 33:83–86.

Meijer, C. J., Rozendaal, L., van der Linden, J. C., Helmerhorst, T. J., Voorhorst, F. J., and Walboomers, J. M. Human papillomavirus testing for primary cervical cancer screening.

Mindel, A., and Carmody, C., Anal human papillomavirus infection. In: Gross, G., and Barrrasso, C., eds., *Human Papillomavirus Infection: A Clinical Atlas.* Ullstein Mosby, 1997.

Moscicki, A. B., Broering, J., Powell, K., et al. Comparison between colposcopic, cytologic, and histologic findings in women positive and negative for human papillomavirus DNA. *J. Adolesc. Health* 1993, 14:74–79.

Moscicki, A. B., Hills, N., Shiboski, S., Powell, K., et al. Risk for incident human papillomavirus infection and low-grade squamous intraepithelial lesion development in young females. *JAMA* 2001, 285:2995–3002.

Moscicki, A. B., Palefsky, J., Gonzales, J., and Schoolnik, G. K. Human papillomavirus infection in sexually active adolescent females: Prevalence and risk factors. *Pediatr. Res.* 1990, 28:507–513.

Moscicki, A. B., Palefsky, J., Smith, G., Siboshski, S., and Schoolnik, G. Variability of human papillomavirus DNA testing in a longitudinal cohort of young women. *Obstet. Gynecol.* 1993, 82:578–585.

Moscicki, A. B., Shiboski, S., Broering, J., et al. The natural history of human papillomavirus infection as measured by repeated DNA testing in adolescent and young women. *J. Pediatr.* 1998, 133:277–284.

Moscicki, A. B., Winkler, B., Irwin, C. E., Jr, and Schachter, J. Differences in biologic maturation, sexual behavior, and sexually transmitted disease between adolescents with and without cervical intraepithelial neoplasia. *J. Pediatr.* 1989, 115:487–493.

Nakagawa, M., Stites, D. P., Farhat, S., et al. T-cell proliferative response to human papillomavirus type 16 peptides: Relationship to cervical intraepithelial neoplasia. *Clin. Diagn. Lab. Immunol.* 1996, 3:205–210.

Nakagawa, M., Stites, D. P., Patel, S., et al. Persistence of human papillomavirus type 16 infection is associated with lack of cytotoxic T lymphocyte response to the E6 antigen. *J. Infect. Dis.* 2000, 182:595–598.

Nash, J., Burke, T., and Hoskins, W. Biologic course of cervical human papillomavirus infection. *Obstet. Gynecol.* 1987, 69:160–162.

National Cancer Institute Workshop. The 1988 Bethesda System for reporting cervical/vaginal cytologic diagnosis. *JAMA* 1989, 262:931–934.

Negangel, C., Munoz, N., Bosch, F. X., et al. The causes of cervical cancer in the Philippines: A case control study. *J. Natl. Cancer Inst.* 1998, 90:43–49.

Nevins, J. R. E2F: A link between the Rb tumor suppressor protein and viral onco-proteins. *Science* 1992, 258:424–429.

Newfield, L., Goldsmith, A., Bradlow, H. L., et al. Estrogen metabolism and human papillomavirus-induced tumors of the larynx: Chemo-prophylaxis with indole-3-carbinol. *Anticancer Research.* 1993, 13:337.

Nobbenhuis, M. A. E., Walboomers, J. M. M., Helmerhorst, T. J. M., Rozendaal, L., et al. Relation of human papillomavirus status to cervical lesions and consequences for cervical screening: A prospective study. *Lancet* 1999, 354:20–25.

Ostor, A. G. Natural history of CIN: A critical review. *Int. J. Gynecol. Pathol.* 1993, 12:186–192

Papillo, J. L., Zarka, M. A., and St. John, T. L. Evaluation of the ThinPrep Pap Test in clinical practice: A seven-month, 16,314-case experience in northern Vermont. *Acta Cytol.* 1998, 42:203–208.

Parrazini, F., Sideri, M., Restelli, S., Schettino, F., Chatenoud, L., and Crosignani, P. G. Determinants of high-grade dysplasia among women with mild dyskaryosis on cervical smear. *Obstet. Gynecol.* 1995, 86:754–757.

Pou, A. M., Rimell, F. L., Jordan, J. A., et al. Adult respiratory papillomatosis: Human papilloma virus (HPV) type and viral coinfections as predictors of prognosis. *Annals Oto., Rhino. Laryng.* 1995, 104:758.

Quick, C. A., Watts, S. L., Krzyzek, R. A., et al. Relationship between condylomata and laryngeal papillomata. *Annals Oto., Rhino. Laryng.* 1980, 89:467.

Raab, S. S., Snider, T. E., Potts, S. A., et al. Atypical glandular cells of undetermined significance: Diagnostic accuracy and interobserver variability using select cytologic criteria. *Am. J. Clin. Pathol.* 1997, 107:299–307.

Remmick, A. J., Walboomers, J. M. M., Helmerhorst, T. J. M., et al. The presence of persistent high-risk HPV genotypes in dysplastic cervical lesions is associated with progressive disease: Natural history up to 36 months. *Int. J. Cancer* 1995, 61:306–311.

Rimell, F. L., Shoemaker, D. L., Pou, A. M., et al. Pediatric respiratory papillomatosis: Prognostic role of viral typing and cofactors. *Laryngoscope.* 1997, 107:915–918.

Robb, J. A. The "ASCUS" swamp. *Diagn. Cytopathol.* 1994, 11:319–320.

Roberts, J. M., Gurley, A. M., Thurloe, J. K., et al. Evaluation of the ThinPrep Pap Test as an adjunct to the conventional Pap smear. *Med. J. Aust.* 1997, 167:460–467.

Roden, R. B., Lowy, D. R., and Schiller, J. T. Papillomavirus is resistant to desiccation. *J. Infect. Dis.* 1997, 176:1076–1079.

Rodriguez, M., Guimares, O., and Rose, P. G. Radical abdominal trachelectomy and pelvic lymphadenectomy with uterine conservation and subsequent pregnancy in the treatment of early invasive cervical cancer. *Am. J. Obstet. Gynecol.* 2001, 185:370–374.

Ronnett, B. M., Manos, M. M., Ransley, J. A., et al. Atypical glandular cells of undetermined significance (AGUS): Cytopathologic features, histopathologic results, and human papillomavirus DNA detection. *Hum. Pathol.* 1999, 30:816–825.

Rosen, C. A., Woodson, G. E., Thompson, J. W., et al. Preliminary results of the use of indole-3-carbinol for recurrent respiratory papillomatosis. *Otolaryng.—Head Neck Surg.* 1998, 118(6):810–815.

Rosenfield, W. D., Vermund, S. H., Wentz, S. J., and Burk, R. D. High prevalence rate of human papillomavirus infection and association with abnormal Papanicolaou smears in sexually active adolescents. *AJDC* 1989, 143:1443–1447.

Rosenthal, D. L. Automation and the endangered future of the Pap test. *J. Nat. Cancer. Inst.* 1998, 90:738–749.

Schachter, J., Hill, E. C., King, E. B., et al. Chlamydia trachomatis and cervical neoplasia. *JAMA* 1982, 248:2134–2138.

Schiffman, M. H., Bauer, H. M., Hoover, R. N., et al. Epidemiologic evidence showing that human papillomavirus infection causes most cervical intraepithelial neoplasia. *J. Natl. Cancer Inst.* 1993, 85:958–964.

Schiffman, M. H., and Brinton, L. A. The epidemiology of cervical carcinogenesis. *Cancer* 1995, 76:1888–1901.

Schiffman, M. H., Haley, N. J., Felton, J. S., et al. Biochemical epidemiology of cervical neoplasia measuring cigarette smoke constituents in the cervix. *Cancer Res.* 1987, 47:3886–3888.

Schiffman, M. H., Manos, M. M., Sherman, M. E., et al. Response: Human papillomavirus and cervical intraepithelial neoplasia. *J. Natl. Cancer Inst.* 1993, 85:1868–1870.

Schiffman, M. H., Solomon, D., Liae, K. L., and Sherman, M. Why, how and when the cytologic diagnosis of ASCUS should be eliminated. *J. Low Tract. Dis.* 1998, 2:165–169.

Schneider, A., Shah, K. The role of vitamins in the etiology of cervical neoplasia: an epidemiological review. *Arch Gynecol Obstet* 1989; 1–13.

Scott, M., Stites, D. P., and Moscicki, A. B. Th1 cytokine patterns in cervical human papillomavirus infection. *Clin. Diagn. Lab Immunol.* 1999, 6:751–755.

Shah, K., Kashima, H. K., Polk, B. F., et al. Rarity of cesarean delivery in cases of juvenile-onset respiratory papillomatosis. *Obst. Gyn.* 1986, 68:795.

Shapiro, A. M., Rimell, F. L., Pou, A., et al. Tracheotomy in children with juvenile-onset recurrent respiratory papillomatosis: The Children's Hospital of Pittsburgh experience. *Annals Otol. Rhino. Laryng.* 1996, 1–5:97–98.

Sherman, M. E., and Kelly, D. High-grade squamous intraepithelial lesions and invasive carcinoma following the report of three negative Papanicolaou smears: Screening failures or rapid progression? *Mod. Pathol.* 1992, 5:337–342.

Sherman, M. E., Schiffman, M. H., and Cox, J. T. The Bethesda System: Biological and clinical correlates. *Pathol. Case Rev.* 1997, 2:3–7.

Sherman, M. E., Schiffman, M., Herrero, R., Kelly, D., Bratti, C., et al. Performance of a semiautomated Papanicolaou smear screening system. *Cancer Cytopathol.* 1998, 84:273–280.

Sherman, M. E., Schiffman, M. H., Lorincz, A. T., et al. Cervical specimens collected in liquid buffer are suitable for both cytologic screening and ancillary human papillomavirus testing. *Cancer Cytopathol.* 1997, 81:89–97.

Sherman, M. E., Schiffman, M. H., Lorincz, A. T., et al. Towards objective quality assurance in cervical cytopathology: Correlation of cytopathologic diagnosis with detection of high risk HPV types. *Am. J. Clin. Pathol.* 1994, 102:182–187.

Sherman, M. E., Schiffman, M. H., Stickler, H., and Hildersheim, A. Prospects for a prophylactic HPV vaccine: Rationale and future implications for cervical cancer screening. *Diagn. Cytopathol.* 1998, 18:5–9.

Slattery, M., Abbott, T., Overall, J., Jr., et al. Dietary vitamins A, C, and E and selenium as risk factors for cervical cancer. *Epid* 1990; 1:8–15.

Solomon, D., Schiffman, M., and Tarone, R. Comparison of three management strategies for patients with atypical squamous cells of undetermined significance: Baseline results from a randomized trial. *J. Natl. Cancer Inst.* 2001, 93:293–299.

Stone, K. M., Zaidi, A., Rosero-Bixby, L., et al. Sexual behavior, sexually transmitted diseases, and risk of cervical cancer. *Epidemiology* 1995, 6:409–414.

Svare, E. I., Kjaer, S. K., Worm, A. M., et al. Risk factors for HPV infection in women from sexually transmitted disease clinics: Comparison between two areas with different cervical cancer incidence. *Intl. J. Cancer* 1998, 75:1–8.

Syrjanen, K. I. Biological behavior of cervical intraepithelial neoplasia. In: Franco, E., and Monsonego, J., eds. *New Developments in Cervical Cancer Screening and Prevention.* London: Blackwell Science, 1997, 93–108.

Tseng, C. J., Liang, C. C., Soong, Y. K., and Pao, C. C. Prenatal transmission of human papillomavirus in infants: Relationship between infection rate and mode of delivery. *Obstet. Gynecol.* 1998, 91:922–996.

Vassilakos, P., Saurel, J., and Rondez, R. Direct-to-vial use of the AutoCyte PREP liquid-based preparations for cervical-vaginal specimens in three European laboratories. *Acta Cytol.* 1999, 43:65–68.

Villa, L. L. Human papillomaviruses and cervical cancer (Review). *Adv. Cancer Res.* 1997, 71:321–341.

Wallin, K.-L., Wiklund, F., Angstrom, T., et al. Type-specific persistence of human papillomavirus DNA before the development of invasive cervical cancer. *N. Engl. J. Med.* 1999, 341:1633–1638.

Werness, B. A., Levine, A. J., and Howley, P. M. Association of human papillomavirus types 16 and 18 E6 proteins with p53. *Science* 1990, 248:76–79.

Wilbur, D. C., Prey, M., Miller, W., Pawlick, G.F., and Colgan, T. J. The AutoPap system for primary screening in cervical cytology. *Acta Cytol.* 1998, 42:214–220.

Winkelstein, W., Jr., Shillitoe, E. J., Brand, R., and Johnson, K. K. Further comments on cancer of the uterine cervix, smoking, and herpes virus infection. *Am. J. Epidemiol.* 1984, 119:1–8.

Wright, T. C., Jr., Is there a role for HPV DNA testing in routine practice? *OBG Man.* 2001.

Wright, T. C., Kurman, R. J., and Ferenczy, A. Precancerous lesions of the cervix. In: Kurman, R. J., ed., *Blaustein's Pathology of the Female Genital Tract.* New York: Springer Verlag, 1995, 248–257.

Wright, T. C., Lorincz, A. T., Ferris, D. G., Richart, R. M., Ferenczy, A., et al. Reflex human papillomavirus deoxyribonucleic acid testing in women with abnormal Pap smears. *Am. J. Obstet. Gynecol.* 1998, 178:962–966.

Wright, T. C., Sun, X. W., and Koulos, J. Comparison of management algorithms for the evaluation of women with low-grade cytologic abnormalities. *Obstet. Gynecol.* 1995, 85:202–210.

Xi, L. F., Koutsky, L. A., Galloway, D. A., Kuypers, J., Hughes, J. P., et al. Genomic variation of human papillomavirus type 16 and risk for high-grade cervical intrae-pithelial neoplasia. *J. Natl. Cancer Inst.* 1997, 89:796–802.

Young, S. Your Pap smear: A save-your-life guide. *Glamour* 1997, 208–211.

Zur Hausen, H. Papillomavirus in anogenital cancer: The dilemma of epidemiologic approaches. *J. Natl. Cancer Inst.* 1989, 81:1680–1682.

Zweizig, S., Noller, K., Reale, F., et al. Neoplasia associated with atypical glandular cells of undetermined significance on cervical cytology. *Gynecol. Oncol.* 1997, 65:314–318.

Resources*

One of the major reasons for this book is to remedy the lack of published material available and oriented to the general public regarding the various diseases caused by HPV infection. Thus an exhaustive list of other published resources isn't possible. There are, however, many excellent general health books and comprehensive women's health books that offer a more in-depth discussion of topics discussed briefly here. A list of these books is provided below.

Golan, Ralph. *Optimal Wellness*. New York: Ballantine, 1995.

Hudson, Tori. *Women's Encyclopedia of Natural Medicine: Alternative Therapies and Integrative Medicine*. Los Angeles: Lowell House, and Chicago: Contemporary Books, 1999.

Linger, Skye W., et al. *The Natural Pharmacy*. Rocklin, CA: Prima Publishing, 1999.

Northrup, Christine. *Women's Body, Women's Wisdom: Creating Physical and Emotional Health and Healing*. New York: Bantam, 1998.

Null, Gary. *The Ultimate Anti-Aging Program*. New York: Keningston, 1999.

Pizzorno, Joseph E. *Total Wellness: Improve Your Health by Understanding the Body's Healing Systems*. Rocklin, CA: Prima Publishing, 1996.

---

*While the author has made every effort to provide accurate telephone numbers and Internet addresses at the time of publication, neither the publisher nor the author assumes any responsibility for errors, or for changes that occur after publication.

Internet-based information and resources greatly outnumber print publications. With the Internet you must consider the source of what you are reading. The Internet sites listed below address many aspects of HPV infection and therapies for the various conditions.

Alliance for Cervical Cancer Prevention   www.alliance-cxca.org

American Academy of Dermatology   http://www.aad.org

American Board of Obstetrics and Gynecology   www.abog.org

American Cancer Society   www.cancer.org

American College of Obstetricians and Gynecologists   www.acog.org

American Holistic Medical Association   www.ahma.org

American Medical Association   http://www.ama-assn.org

American Society for Colposcopy and Cervical Pathology   http://www.asccp.org

Center for Cervical Health   www.cervicalhealth.org

Centers for Disease Control and Prevention   www.cdc.gov/std

Digene-HPV Information, Hybrid Capture II   www.digene.com

Digene-Women's Health   www.digene.com

Family Health International   www.fhi.org

A Forum for Women's Health   www.womenshealth.org

The HPV Test   www.thehpvtest.com

International Papillomavirus Society   www.ipvsoc.org

JAMA Women's Health   www.ama-assn.org/special/std/std.htm

National Breast and Cervical Cancer Early Detection Program
www.cdcc.gov/cancer/nbccedp/index.htm

National Cervical Cancer Coalition   www.nccc-online.org

National Cervical Cancer Public Education Campaign
http://www.cervicalcancercampaign.org

National Institutes of Health   http://www.nih.gov

National Women's Health Information Center   www.4women.org

National Women's Health Resource Center   www.healthywomen.org

Nutritional Information   www.mercola.com

OBGYN.net   www.obgyn.net

The Respiratory Papillomavirus Home Page   www.rrpf.org

ThinPrep Pap Test—Woman's Health Center, Cytyc Corporation
www.thinprep.com

3M Pharmaceuticals-Aldara (Imiquimod)   3m.com/us/healthcare/pharma

Women for HPV Testing   www.womenforhpvtesting.org/index.html

Women's Cancer Network   http://www.wen.org

Women's Health Interactive   http://www.womens-health.com

World Health Organization   www.who.int/home-page

I can offer myself, my partners, and our excellent staff as a resource for additional information. In many cases we may be able to refer you to local physicians to provide you with the information and care you need. You may also contact us for information about the HPV Foundation. Our address is:

Gregory S. Henderson, M.D., Ph.D.
Women's Diagnostic Division
Wilmington Pathology Associates, P.A.
2106 South 17th Street
Wilmington, NC 28401
E-mail: Dr.Henderson@HPVFoundation.org

Index

About the Authors

GREGORY STEPHEN HENDERSON, M.D., PH.D., attended Vanderbilt University as a National Institute of Health Medical Scientist Training Program Fellow, where he received his medical degree and a Ph.D. in immunology. He is certified by the American Board of Pathology and is a Fellow of the College of American Pathology. Dr. Henderson is the director of The Wilmington Pathology Associates, P.A.'s Women's Diagnostic Division, Chairman of the Department of Pathology at New Hanover Regional Medical Center, and a Clinical Assistant Professor in the Department of Surgery at the University of North Carolina School of Medicine. He lives in Wilmington, North Carolina, with his wife, Isabelle, and his daughters, Margaux and Ava.

BATYA SWIFT YASGUR, M.A., MSW, is a freelance writer. She earned a Master's degree in Near Eastern Languages from Harvard University and a Master's of Social Work from Rutgers University. She is a regular contributor to *Clinical Psychiatry News*, *Pediatric News,* and *Ob/Gyn News*, and is the author of *Keep It Fresh, Good-Bye Diapers*, and *America: A Freedom Country*.

ALLAN WARSHOWSKY, M.D., is an obstetrician/gynecologist and the Director of the Women's Program of the Continuum Center for Health and Healing at Beth Israel Hospital in Manhattan. His practice therapies range from conventional to purely holistic, including such modalities as nutritional therapy, herbal treatments, and lifestyle management, as well as visualization, imagery, and other stress-reduction techniques.